LAUGHING IN THE FACE OF CANCER

ALSO BY PAM LACKO

"Prescription: Humor " (essay)

LAUGHING IN THE FACE OF CANCER

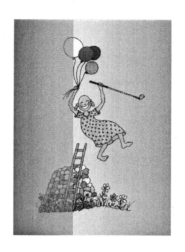

by Pam L

A

Simsb

and Sarah McQuilkin

ark Lacko

cQuilkin

ast.net
oks.com

This book is dedicated to the two people who saw me through my toughest times battling cancer. The first is my husband, Jeff, who put up with every quick decision I made about getting body parts removed, told me how good I looked bald, and took care of our children and the day-to-day activities that allowed our family to feel normal during a very abnormal time. The second is my mother, Theresa, who was my rock, escorting me to every appointment, blood test, CAT Scan, MRI, and treatment. She is the best advocate a person can have and a pillar of strength.

ACKNOWLEDGEMENTS

Many friends have helped me through my battle with Cancer or through my efforts to translate that battle into words. I thank you all and especially the following:

Molly Brewer, D.V.M., M.D., M.S.; Lori Wilson, M.D., F.A.C.S.; Jonathan Schrieber, M.D.; Robin Schwartz M.S., C.G.C.; Andre Kaplan, M.D.; Cheryl Vincent, D.C.; Rebecca Huntley, L.M.T.; Carm Natelli, R.N.; Jen Stapell, R.N.; Kristie Dubey, R.N.; Kristie Michaud, R.N.; Bernie Siegel, M.D.; Michelle Twigg, M.D.; Linda Lightner, Rennie McQuilkin, Sarah McQuilkin, and Donna Collins.

To that list I'd like to add the entire medical staff at the Carole and Ray Neag Comprehensive Cancer Center of The University of Connecticut, and in particular the nurses and staff of the 6th floor at the Center.

Last and far from least, I am forever grateful to all of my family members, clients and colleagues who lent their support during my hazardous journey. Rebecca and Mathew, you were an ultimate life support system. Thank you for tolerating my mood swings, for providing many hugs, and for the extra care you showed me.

TABLE OF CONTENTS

FOREWORD

It's terribly annoying to pee every ten minutes and even more annoying when you're not at home. Looking back at it all now, I see that I knew something was wrong in September of 2007. I even mentioned it to my trainer at the gym. I felt bloated, had gained weight when I was working out four or five days a week and eating "right." I thought it might be my thyroid medication (sometimes you can lose weight when your thyroid medication is upped—anything to avoid dieting) and was disappointed to find that my thyroid levels were well within the normal range. The pieces wouldn't really come together until February of 2008 when I was diagnosed with Stage IIB Ovarian Cancer.

LAUGHING IN THE FACE OF CANCER

CHAPTER ONE: SYMPTOMS

Gotta Go Right Now!

During the holidays we visit family in New York and inevitably end up at the local mall. My two kids, niece, sister in law, and I all head off to return gifts and shop for post-holiday sales. In 2007 it was the week between Christmas and New Years. We were all dressed in heavy clothing, so going to the bathroom was something to do sparingly.

Minutes into our shopping excursion, I was in a return merchandise line at American Eagle with my sister in law when I started doing the shaking of the leg dance. The shaking turned to tapping my foot and a subtle swaying. Well, it didn't take long for me to excuse myself from the line and walk as fast as I could, keeping my legs together as tightly as possible, to find a restroom. Wandering aimlessly in an unfamiliar mall was bad enough, but having the urge to pee like a horse was over the top. It was then that I knew some woman would make millions if she could invent a handheld GPS that could detect and direct you to the nearest ladies room.

My sister in law caught up to me and told me to go into Macy's, where there was a restroom near the Customer Service Dept. At this point my dance had turned into a shuffle. I couldn't increase my stride, fearing I might spring a leak. I'm sure it was obvious to any other woman in the store that I had to go. We all do the same dance you know.

It's funny that when you know relief is near the urge to go gets even stronger. So there I was, standing in front of three stalls in the ladies room, all with women in them. Now I was doing the dance much more outwardly, relieved to be in the privacy of a restroom. It felt like forever as I waited to hear a familiar flush and the click of a door being unlocked. All I could wonder was "What happens if I can't make it? I guess I could go buy some new underwear and jeans and just meet up with the others later in the day and tell them I'd lost the jeans I'd come in." Finally, someone was finishing up. Again, I felt another surge of pressure on my bladder, knowing relief was near. The door flew open and I immediately headed into the stall, practically knocking down the woman exiting. Now the sensation was so intense it was painful.

Looking down, I realize I still have a long road ahead of me. I take off my ski jacket as I clench my legs tightly together in the stall, pivoting only to find that the hook on the door has been removed. "Damn it," I say aloud. I'm not going to put my jacket on the floor, so I put it back on. Now I find myself humming along with the dancing to keep my mind off wetting myself. Under my sweater I feel for my button and zipper and realize that I have worn a belt today. "Damn it," I say again. Out of all days, why in hell did I wear a belt? More dancing and swaying. (Boy, if anyone has been outside the stall watching my feet this whole time, they must be wondering what in God's name I'm doing). Anyway, I get the belt undone, unbutton my pants, pull down my zipper, and look down at that public toilet. The big question in my mind is, "Can I hover over the bowl while holding my clothing out of the way without missing?" At this point I am ready to bust so I just take my best shot even though I can't see a thing from the front with my ski jacket and sweater in the way, never mind trying to look over my bloated stomach.

It's amazing how women know how to pee in the worst of places and can adjust while in the squatting position to make sure we don't miss. Just by the shear sound of the event we can move our butts ever so slightly to the left or right so we can achieve a direct hit.

As soon as I was done, I hiked up my jeans, closed everything up, latched my belt and flushed the toilet. Guess what—I felt the urge again. How frustrating was that! Off with the belt, down with the jeans and so on. I eventually had a spell when I felt somewhat normal, caught up to my shopping group and headed back to the stores, cautiously optimistic that I could make it the rest of the afternoon if I didn't have anything to drink.

Needless to say this was embarrassing to my kids, and it was obvious to my sister in law that something was wrong. She suggested that I go to the walk-in clinic to see if I had a bladder infection. So when we returned to Connecticut on New Years Eve, I did just that. The doctor there confirmed that I did not have an infection but thought I had an "overactive bladder." He prescribed Detrol and said that if it didn't resolve the issue, I should see my general physician. Luckily my annual physical was scheduled for January 9th, so I took Detrol as prescribed over the next ten days. By the 9th I still felt no relief, so I mentioned the issue to my GP during my appointment.

She examined me and said that I should make an appointment with my OBGYN because the female organs near the bladder might be causing the problem. When I called my OBGYN's office, I learned that the earliest they could see me was March 4th. I said ok, not thinking it was an urgent issue; and let's face it—by now I was getting pretty used to frequent stops in the ladies' room. It's amazing what we can tolerate. At this point I wasn't concerned about my later-to-be-discovered issue, but was concentrating on how I could be the woman to invent the "LRL" or Ladies' Room Locator.

I had planned a week's vacation in mid-January to visit my mother in Florida. By then I was very uncomfortable, peeing like a horse and having abdominal pain when doing my sit-ups. I also had break-through bleeding between periods. Most of this could be attributed to the onset of menopause, so I would wait to talk to my OBGYN.

When I got back to Connecticut and told a friend about my problem, I swear she saved my life. She told me to hang up the phone, call my OBGYN's office, and demand to be seen right away. What a smart friend! They got me in the next day, did five biopsies of my cervix and sent me for an Ultra Sound of my ovaries. By the way, this was the second time I'd gone to an appointment by myself and ended up having biopsies performed. Don't go to appointments alone. Biopsies suck! Actually they hurt *and* suck!

The OBGYN found the problem. One ovary was the size of a grapefruit and the other was a golf ball. Apparently ovaries are supposed to be the size of apricots. Who comes up with these sizing analogies anyway?

Given the fact that my grandmother died of Ovarian Cancer at the young age of 47, I was referred to the OBGYN Oncology Department for a consultation. My husband and I spent forty-five minutes the next Monday with Dr. Molly Brewer, who would become my surgeon, my oncologist, my gynecologist, and the doctor who saved my life. My surgery was scheduled for Thursday that same week. That was February 4th, 2008. Thank goodness I wasn't going to need that Ladies' Room Locator any longer. Soon, I would be peeing normally again, or at least that's what I thought!

Chapter Two: My Hospital Stay

Going into my surgery, I was told that if they were able to just take the ovaries through a laparoscopic procedure, then I would be home the same day. If not, I would go home the next day. Five days later, I was released from the hospital. But in my five days there, I had three experiences that were comical to look back on. Here are those stories.

The Laptop Story (Always Marketing the Business)

As my husband Jeff and I sat in our pre-op corner of the Procedure Center at the hospital, we read the newspaper, joked about the surgery, and waited patiently for an operating room to become available. After a while, a very young and good-looking doctor walked in and said that he would be my anesthesiologist for the procedure and that his boss would be sitting in as well.

His boss showed up in a couple of minutes, angry at his swivel-top laptop. He apologized and said that he couldn't start my surgery until he fixed the laptop so that he could print out my history at the main desk. Well, I saw my opportunity and grabbed it.

"My husband and I run a computer-consulting business, so maybe we can help," I said. Quickly, Jeff took a look, tried a couple of remedies, and sure enough, was able to resolve the problem twenty minutes into my scheduled surgery time. The doctor was thrilled, but said he couldn't deduct any of the cost. He did add that he lived in West Simsbury and would love it if we could help him out with his home computers. He smiled at me as he put me to sleep! I have forgotten his name, and I'm sure he doesn't remember mine. Oh well.

Extreme Makeover and the Crucifixion

My operation was originally scheduled for 9:30 a.m. on a Thursday morning, but several things, including fixing the anesthesiologist's laptop, delayed it until about 11:00. As Jeff and I sat in the pre-op area, my doctor came in and said she had finished her first surgery (glad she practiced before mine), and had to check on her patient. She said they were fixing up the operating room and we'd be delayed about an hour.

Fifteen minutes later, one of the residents who would be "scrubbing in" on the surgery (happy they wash their hands), said they were almost through getting the operating room all done up and she'd be back to get me in a bit.

Moments later, another resident stopped in and said exactly the same thing, so I was thinking that this operating room was going to be one spiffy space.

During a surgery in 2001 at another local hospital, I remember being "drugged" in the pre-op area. I assumed they did this so the patient wouldn't have any fears going into the operating room. Apparently I didn't need it today or they didn't think I would care when I actually saw the operating room in the condition it was in. Whoa.

They rolled me into a tiny, drably grey space that looked nothing like an operating room except for the big lights overhead. I asked why they had brought me into this closet, and the residents (laughing of course) said, "Oh no, Mrs. Lacko, this is your operating room," to which I answered, "You all told me you were working hard to get the room ready. I was expecting something a bit more...colorful." Frank, the designer from Trading Spaces, must have done this room. Yuk. No extreme make-over here.

To my right was a stainless steel table about eight inches in width. I looked around as best as I could to see where the operating table was, but lo and behold, that was the only one in the room. They rolled my gurney next to this pencil-thin table. "That's not the operating table is it?" I asked. "I couldn't possibly fit my entire body on that."

"No problem," one resident said as they lifted my sheet and my butt off the gurney and placed me back-end down on the shiny sliver. Needless to say, I didn't budge. Adjusting my Johnny at this point would have cost me dearly—with a face plant on the floor.

The anesthesiologist then tried to keep my mind off what he was about to do, talking about the weather and the food in the cafeteria. As he was keeping me occupied (that's what he thought), he asked me to put out my left arm and pulled out a neat little stainless steel wing from the table, immediately strapping my arm down and attaching assorted monitoring devices, all the while talking casually about life.

Then he whipped out another one of those wings, asked for my other arm, and strapped *it* down. I'd thought I was doing pretty well, cracking some jokes and humoring him with responses to his cafeteria stories. But now I was beginning to feel like one of those squirrels that has fallen off an electrical power line and landed on its back, eyes wide open, in the middle of the street.

Last, but certainly not least, a nurse came out with a ten-inch leather strap and connected it to one side of the table, up and over my thighs, and snapped it to the other side of the table. I lay there thinking *This isn't going to be the "internal laparoscopic procedure" I had in mind.* By now they had pretty much blocked off any optical access to my ovaries.

So, as we approached Good Friday, I was pretty sure I'd come dangerously close to feeling like Jesus on the cross. Next time I would bring my own table!

My Ball and Chain

After surgery and time in the recovery room, they moved me to a semi-private room up on the sixth floor. I was a bit out of it but did realize that I had a roommate. I swear I must have kept her up all night whining about my pain. Fortunately for her, she was discharged the next morning. My stay was private from that point on.

I woke up on Friday morning to find that my "Johnny" was all wet in the front. This was odd, as I had a catheter in, and anyway I was pretty sure a woman can't pee forward. I buzzed for the nurse and had her check it out. She thought that my "pain booster" or my incision might be leaking. Great, I thought. I didn't even know I had a "pain booster." Just what I needed!

They sent in a resident to check it out. A tall blonde named Dr. Sing (I've changed her name to protect the innocent). She was really nervous and unsure of herself as she poked at my stomach. I was getting a little nervous too. I told her that if she wasn't sure what was wrong, she didn't have to touch the trouble spot. I didn't mind being wet, I told her.

She checked with the doctor and came back to say that my "pain booster" might be leaking a bit, but the doctor wanted to keep it in. What was this "pain booster" thing she was talking about? I couldn't budge my head enough to see what was on my stomach, so the mystery continued.

That afternoon they took out the catheter and said I should get up to pee. Yeh right. Getting up was hard enough, never mind walking over to that bathroom halfway across Connecticut.

With help from my nurse, I sat up and was immediately drawn back down to the pillow by some weight in the bed. When the nurse asked, "What's wrong?" I said, "Something is dragging me under." We looked under the sheets and found a ball about the size of a large Christmas ornament with a tube leading under my Johnny. "Oh, this must be the pain booster," said my knowledgeable nurse. "I've never actually seen one of these before."

Great, I thought. Dr. Sing is jittery, and my knowledgeable nurse just found out what a "pain booster" looks like. I'm in good hands here!

I figured out that in order for me to move anywhere, my ornament must come with me. When I picked it up, I realized it weighed two or three pounds, which felt more like ten at the time. So with my right hand on my moving drug cart and the ball in my left hand, I was escorted to the bathroom miles away with my backside showing to the whole sixth floor. *Hey,* I thought, *if people think my backside is bad, they should take a look at my front!*

When I got to the throne, I again realized something troubling. The amount of tubing connecting me to the ball was only about eight inches long. This wasn't nearly enough line to set the ball on the floor while peeing. So what was a girl to do? Pee one handed was my Day One answer.

On Day Two I got smarter. While I was sitting there holding my ball and chain, I saw a paper bag hanging from the wall next to the toilet. Though it was a small bag, I thought it was big enough to hold my ball. But was it strong enough? I couldn't quite reach the bag, so I tossed my ball in, risking my life—if the ball made the bag fall to the ground, I would be pulled off the toilet. The bag held tight. I called my nurse in and told her I had found a ball-holder. She immediately reinforced the bag by putting more tape on the wall and patted me on the back for being so creative. I was feeling pretty proud of myself at that point.

CHAPTER THREE: STARTING TREATMENT

The C Word

Cancer. Not what I was hoping to hear and worse, not Stage I but Stage II. I would require chemotherapy. Chemo is such an intimidating word. *Will I lose my hair? What do I do about my business, my drum students, time with my family this spring and summer? How sick will I get? Will the chemo actually work or is this the end?* All these questions ran through my mind.

To answer these questions and more, we needed a plan for our next appointment with Dr. Brewer. So I called a family meeting. Luckily we have a small family, so we could easily fit around the game table in our family room. Sitting with my laptop in front of me, I documented every question on my mind, my sister's, my mother's and my husband's. I should have included my kids, but didn't think about it at the time. I guess I was trying to keep them safe from this for now. Everyone had different concerns about me and about my future. It was an interesting process. Whereas I was worried about my chances of surviving, my husband wanted to know if I could still have cheese and crackers with wine. Anyway, we compiled a list of forty-two questions which we brought to my appointment. My mother, my husband and I sat there with Dr. Brewer for a good hour, listening and taking copious notes on all her answers.

Now armed with this information, I felt that there wouldn't be any surprises over the next six months. I felt empowered with the knowledge of what was to come, and my family members felt that their questions and concerns had been addressed.

Meet Dixie

In that follow-up visit with my oncologist, I learned that I would need six chemotherapy treatments to ensure they got all of the cancer. I asked what the side-effects were, and she said that everyone was different but that one side effect was certain: I would lose my hair, all of my hair, everywhere and soon after my first treatment.

With that information, I went home, called three of my wacky and close friends, and arranged a shopping trip to a large wig store in the area. Shopping would be followed by a full-course breakfast at a local diner. Excellent eggs! Gotta bulk up for chemo!

When we all arrived, the store was empty of customers. Thank goodness for that. We are loud and obnoxious when we get laughing and that's exactly what we did. There were hundreds of wigs of all sizes, shapes, colors and lengths. My nutty friends went for the pink and purple models, while the more mature side of the room, I myself, went for exactly what I would sport for months.

So we came down to two wigs, Amanda and Dixie Pixie. I didn't realize at the time that the wigs had names—I was shopping for the right look, not the name. When the salesperson showed me the name on the tag of the one I favored, the decision was a no-brainer. Dixie Pixie was for me.

It's Raining Hair

It was a morning about six days after my first chemotherapy treatment when I noticed some short blonde hairs on my pillow, and when I combed my hair after showering, there were lots more in the comb. I waited until 9:00 a.m. and called my hairdresser to tell her it was starting. She was all prepared. Two weeks before she had cut/trimmed my new wig (they come really thick so she'd thinned it out a bit) and was ready to take me on a moment's notice to shave my head once my hair started coming out in clumps.

My son had told me that he would buzz his hair with me the day I did mine so I wouldn't be bald alone. He was twelve at the time. My fifteen-year-old year daughter offered to get a trim and highlights, a sufficient sacrifice, she thought, one that would make me feel better. I laughed and told Matt that I would take him up on his offer.

On the morning of the "clumping," I had a meeting first thing at our local Chamber of Commerce. Although a few people around the table knew my situation, not everyone did, though I had never worn a baseball cap during a meeting before. Unfortunately, that morning the largest clump of hair had come out just where the baseball hat had a hole in the back. (Why do they make that hole there anyway?) So it was pretty obvious to anyone at the table that I was losing my hair. My white skin and weakness might have tipped them off too.

I went from the meeting to the school to get Matt and then directly to the hairdresser. I had Dixie with me in her box and was ready to leave the salon with her in place. I sat in the chair with my back to the mirror as Donna, my hairdresser, buzzed off the rest of the 'do. Mathew looked on with his mouth gaping open as the little hair I had left dropped to the floor. I had Donna put the wig on and then it was Matt's turn. No big deal for him, but I gave him the same gaping look just to make light of the situation. I didn't look in the mirror until later that night. I looked pretty damn good bald!

Dixie's First Bath

I was told when I bought Dixie that she would need a shampooing in two weeks. So exactly two weeks after I started to wear her, I decided it was time. I did her on Friday night, to be sure my hairdresser would be working the next day—just in case.

Dixie was submerged in cold water, cleansed with a special

shampoo and conditioner, then placed on her drying rack (yes they actually have a special drying rack for wigs) for the evening. To be honest, she looked like a dead rat. I went to bed very nervous that evening.

When I awoke Saturday morning, I ran downstairs to the rack where Dixie had spent the night and was surprised to see her still looking like a dead rat, though a dry one. The next step was to style her. I had two choices: style her on my head, or style her on her normal sleeping place, the white mannequin head that held her when she was off duty.

I chose to style her on my head and found that when you brush a wig, it just comes right off. After a few drops to the floor, I got the hang of holding the wig down with one hand and brushing gently with the other. After my experience in the hospital with the ball and chain, I felt confident that I could master styling my hair one-handed.

The wig came out great. I did not need to have it professionally styled, and I even stopped in to show my hairdresser, who was quite impressed with the result. Another experience behind me and I was feeling good!

My "Red Bull"

The family and I took a vacation over the April school break, now that three of my six chemo treatments were behind me. We flew to Florida, golf clubs in tow, and landed at my mom's beautiful winter home in Siesta Key. For me, it was fabulous to be away from doctors and treatment rooms, so I took every advantage of my reprieve. I did have to get blood work done each Friday to make sure my counts were normal, but other than that I was free of the hospital.

After golfing a few days, playing tennis and swimming, my son and I were just about to tee off on the first of another eighteen holes when my cell phone rang. It was my nurse from the hospital.

She sounded concerned: "How are you feeling?" I answered, mimicking her voice, "I'm fine, how are you?" Her answer was to state that my red blood count was drastically low and that I should be feeling very fatigued. I told her I felt fine and had been swimming, playing golf, and batting the tennis ball around. She was surprised, to say the least, and thought maybe she had received someone else's blood results. We agreed that I would re-take the blood test and that she would call back in two days.

I hung up the phone and proceeded to hit a six iron to the green: a great start. But by the thirteenth hole my game had gone down the drain. I had lost six balls, one of which was at least two streets away after a hooked drive off the tenth tee. Now I started to wonder whether the nurse was right after all. Maybe I could blame my red blood cells for my elevated score.

My second blood test yielded the same results, so when I got home from Florida two days later, I was scheduled for my first blood transfusion at the hospital. After an hour and three separate nurses, someone finally found a vein and started the infusion. What a shot of Red Bull. It's amazing how quickly you notice a difference after a transfusion. The only complaint (aside from the poking to find a vein) was that after I got the blood, my stomach felt a bit unsettled. I guess the blood had come from someone whose lunch hadn't agreed with him or her.

So if you ever need blood, make sure you ask for a donor who has had a balanced meal of something you like too!

A New Bird Sighting

As a result of a friend's advice, I started doing acupuncture and massage to minimize the side-effects of chemo treatments. But what to do to develop more accessible veins? For me, the hardest part of getting treatment was getting the needle in the vein. Yes I am a whimp, but my veins are not cooperative either. Each treatment took multiple nurses and three or four tries to find a friendly vein. It was not only painful, but time-consuming. Each treatment took about six hours, and the vein problem added another hour or two. So I began by asking everyone I knew (including my acupuncture specialist, my massage therapist, my nurses, doctors, postman, and garbage man) what I could do to improve my veins.

The feedback was this: drink a lot of water before your appointment, perform three hundred bicep curls daily for a week, and circle your arms right before you go into the treatment room to get blood flowing to the veins. So the next day I combined all of these tricks, starting in the parking lot straight through to the treatment room. If asked, I was prepared to let those in the waiting room know that there was a new and exotic bird in Connecticut which flapped and pulsed and drank heavily.

You're So "Vein"

My veins continued to be problematic each time I went for my treatments. It became very painful and frustrating for everyone involved. In addition, each time the nurses eventually locked into a vein, the days following treatment were painful for the arm they had used. The veins discolored, my arm swelled, and it was painful to the touch. How was I supposed to know that the "poison" they administered to fix the cancer would make me unable to lift a glass of wine?

After my fourth treatment, I figured I would be really active and keep my mind off my body aches. So I golfed on Tuesday and again on Wednesday. By Wednesday evening I couldn't move my discolored and aching left arm. I decided to call the head oncology nurse and tell her what was going on. She flipped and said I should have told someone I was having this type of reaction each time.

The upshot was that I was told my veins were toast—I would need a "port." I was going to call this article "I prefer Chardonnay over Port," but someone said people might not get it.

I had two treatments to go, so the port would be surgically

implanted on May 22nd and I would get my chemo immediately following the same day. The irony in it all was that in order for me to get my Port, the anesthesiologist would need to find a vein to put me to sleep. This would be interesting, I thought.

Maybe the anesthesiologist would be the one who had developed laptop problems during my first surgery. This time I'd bring my business card. They ought to make Johnnies with pockets.

Going Out for Eighteen Holes

No, I'm not talking about my new favorite sport, golf. Acupuncture had become my latest best friend. Almost weekly since March I'd been seeing Dr. Cheryl, who was fantastic both as a doctor and as a person. She's made a hole-in-one each time.

At my first appointment, she gently took my wrist and held her fingers on my pulse for quite awhile. She said she was "seeing how my rivers flowed." I actually thought she might have dozed off there for a few minutes. I didn't know I had rivers flowing and told her it was probably a "raging stream" due to my Type A personality. She agreed and starting talking about "meridians" and "chi " and all this Chinese stuff I didn't really understand, but it sounded cool.

Considering my issues with needles, I'm sure you are surprised that I even chose to go down this path, but a good friend of mine had told me acupuncture helped her through chemo. "Why not?" I said.

I found out the hard way during one appointment that once the needle is in, you should not move or flex your muscles. Ouch! And don't let your nose itch or curl your toes while lying there with two-inch metal pins sticking out of your body. I also learned that my right ear doesn't like to have a needle in it very long. As soon as Dr. Cheryl left the room, *pop*—it jumped right out. Rejected.

Still, between acupuncture and the "Hot Stone Massages" I

had also begun, I not only felt better but much pampered by these highly trained professionals. Maybe someone will come up with a combination of the two called "AcuStoneMassage".

My Designated Drivers

It happened again. Gene called from the hospital yesterday and said my counts were low. "How low?" I asked. "Really low, like you can't drive yourself to the hospital for the blood transfusion and you can't drive at all until you get blood," she said. So for the rest of the day my husband drove me around town, and then my mother became my "designated driver" to and from my blood transfusion. Timing was everything. The next morning I would be playing golf with my friend Laurie and would be able to hit the ball a ton, considering my new and improved blood supply. There was definitely an advantage to some of this!

What Do You Know, It's Vertigo

Another battle was yet to come. I went to the Talcott Music Festival on Friday, July 11th, to see their tribute to Motown. There were seventeen of us with lots of food, wine and good conversation. I thought the concert was outstanding, but when it was over I was a bit dizzy. No, really dizzy, not my usual dizzy!

I brushed it off, thinking I might have had more glasses of wine than I should have, but on Saturday the dizziness got worse and worse as the day went on. In addition, I got violently sick to my stomach, and I went downhill from there. Sunday morning I was in the ER with low to no electrolytes and severe nausea. They sent me for a brain CAT Scan, which came back normal (see, I *am* somewhat normal) and said the problem was probably Vertigo. Nine hours and seven bags of fluids later, I was still dizzy.

So up I went to the 6th floor (the oncology floor where I first experienced my "ball and chain"). I recognized one of the nurses, who assured me she would take good care of me. I got into my private room (a luxury of chance, it being the only room available) and proceeded to ask for my anti-nausea medication. My caring nurse said NO. "No?" I said. She said that the Zofran they were giving me was the reason for my headache and put a patch behind my ear that would last for three days. Apparently people use them for sea sickness. Well, I guess she knew what she was talking about because the nausea subsided and the headache went away within an hour.

I stayed in the hospital until Tuesday afternoon, getting better each day. Once back home, I couldn't yet function completely on my own but worked over the phone with clients and even had my mother take me to a client—the designated driver scenario once again!

All in all, Vertigo was quite an inconvenience, and I must say it really screwed up my golf game. At the same time this was happening, one of our golden retrievers, Bree, scratched the side of her face so badly she had to go on Prednisone and an antibiotic. She had the infamous lampshade on her head, and between the two of us walking into walls, we kept Jeff and kids quite busy. (As some of you know, Bree loves playing ball. Now when she brought us a ball in her mouth, she looked like a lamp with a bulb in it)

"Stop That—I Barely Know You!"

When I was in the hospital with vertigo, results of my CAT Scan from the prior week had come back and showed spots on my liver. Although they were likely cysts, my very conservative doctor ordered an MRI to get a better diagnosis. Well, that was about enough to send me off the deep end. An MRI. Lovely.

They had one MRI machine at the hospital and it was extremely busy all of the time. My appointment was scheduled for 9:30 p.m. on a Thursday evening. Yes, I said 9:30 *p.m.* Luckily I didn't need to fast, so that wasn't an issue. My trusted driver, Mother Theresa, came to get me at 8:45 p.m. and off we went. I had just gotten out of the hospital on Tuesday, so my Vertigo was still severe. I was, however, wearing a medication patch behind my ear for nausea, but I was still very unsteady on my feet.

Being a proud person, I wouldn't let my mother get me a wheelchair for the walk to the MRI department, so she dropped me off out in front of the hospital, and I held up the building until she came to escort me in. During my walk, I held onto every bit of wall and my mother's arm. It took all of my strength just to focus on putting one foot in front of the other. Sometimes I would see eight feet. Not good, I thought.

So we got down to the MRI department and noticed that it was "under construction." A sign read, "Please report to the Imaging Department." Well, we turned around and walked back the way we'd come (I fondling the wall as I went) and down to the Imaging Department. After about fifteen minutes, the lady behind the desk said, "Oh, they are ready for you now." Back up I got and gathered all of my strength for another long walk back to the construction zone.

Once there, we waited until a technician wearing "Cindy" on her chest came out of the Exit door. Cindy said, "Follow me" as she pranced out the Exit door into the warm night and down a very intimidating metal ramp. "Excuse me...Cindy? I need some help here. You see, I have Vertigo and I see two of you on the ramp. I'm not sure which one is the real you. Can you take my arm and help me?" Cindy did her duty, helping me down the ramp and up the narrow stairs to what looked like a small mobile home—the MRI trailer. Meanwhile, mom sat patiently in the only chair outside the Exit door of the "construction zone." I hoped she'd be ok. Once in the trailer I said to Cindy, "I have a port in my chest that was accessed this afternoon so you could shoot the contrast [dye] in it for the MRI. The veins in my arms are fried from the chemo, so my doctor called ahead of time to let you know about the port." Cindy looked concerned and blurted "WE DON'T DO MRIs

WITH PORTS." That's when I said, "Look Cindy, it's ten o'clock on a Thursday evening. I have severe Vertigo; I have been treated for Ovarian Cancer for the past seven months; and now my doctor says that my CAT Scan shows spots on my liver and that an MRI is the only thing that will tell them what the spots are for sure. So we're going to do this MRI somehow, some way, and it's going to be tonight!"

Todd, another technician who was using a nearby phone, overheard the discussion I was having with Cindy and interjected "Oh, I've seen this done at another hospital. I know how to do it." Great, I thought. He's seen it done. *Well,* I thought, *this is the teaching hospital. Let's teach Cindy how to do an MRI with contrast through a port; and Todd, who has seen it done, can be the teacher. I'm game!*

So while Todd ran off to find some "extension tubing" for my port, Cindy proceeded to get me ready on the MRI table and let me know that if she had used the pump to put the contrast into my port, I would have died on the table. Cindy needs to work on her bedside manner.

So here's the scenario. I'm lying on my back on the MRI table. I will go into the machine head first and nothing will be sticking out. My port is just above my left breast and has about three inches of tubing sticking out of it. Todd now attaches the extension tubing, which snakes around to about mid-thigh. Todd explains that the first part of the test does not include the contrast and that he will let me know when he comes in to inject it manually (so I won't die on the table). Wouldn't that be a hoot—to die from dye!

At this point Cindy offers me headphones and asks if I would like to listen to 100.5's easy listening music. "Sure," I said. Here I go. The table is moving now into the machine, and as I look at how close the machine is to my face and body I start to think *This isn't going to pleasant at all.*

I felt like a sausage being put into its casing and decided to close my eyes the entire time (I would recommend this to anyone having an MRI) while visualizing a round of golf. It worked. I was calm, cool, and collected during the procedure, which lasted a full hour. By the way, I didn't play the course well and still sliced my drives almost every hole.

When it was time for the contrast, Todd said (I could hear him in my headphones), "I'm coming in to inject the contrast." "Ok," I said. Thirty seconds later I felt a hand going up my leg. "Mrs. Lacko, it's only me, Todd. I'm trying to find the end of the extension tubing." I responded, "Todd, I just met you, and I think you might be overstepping your technician authority right now. The extension tubing is on the other thigh. Please be quick, I barely know you."

When it was all said and done, I learned that my mother, waiting patiently, had been my advocate out in that little construction zone called her waiting room. When Todd had passed her while looking for the extension tubing, he'd said, "We need to run an IV line," to which mom had answered, "ABSOLUTELY NOT. NO ONE TOUCHES HER VEINS. USE THE PORT!" Go, Mom.

It's Good To Be Negative

Now I'm not a negative person. But there's something to be said for negativity. My good friend Mary Beth, who lived with Ovarian Cancer for almost seven years, used to ask me, "So when is a negative a positive?" I never really got the impact of that question and the answer until today.

I learned the answer while sitting at home, hoping that the phone would ring with good news. At 5:00 p.m. my nurse from the hospital called to say the MRI was NEGATIVE. Phew.

So now I could focus on growing my hair back and not worrying about more treatments. I had been watering my head daily and using Miracle Grow once a week. Nothing yet. I was beginning to think I might be seen on the Chia Pet commercial when they started advertising again for the holidays.

Mother Theresa

I have mentioned my mother in this book many times and some-times have referred to her as Mother Theresa. Although I go to a Christian church every Sunday, I wouldn't say that I am an overly religious individual. I was born and raised Catholic, went to cat-echism classes, and was confirmed and eventually married in a Catholic church. But I need to clarify why I refer to my mom as Mother Theresa.

It's true that my mom was one of my two health advocates (the other being my husband, Jeff) and accompanied me to many of my appointments, treatments and tests. She guided me to my MRI when I had severe Vertigo. As I've said, she fought with a technician who tried to access a vein in my arm (don't get her mad). She reminded me (and still does) to take my medications when I traveled and to schedule my routine blood work. She was attentive when I mentioned an ache or a pain and was as well informed and concerned about my treatment and test results as if it had been her own health on the line. I did think of her as a Saint, and still do, but the primary reason I refer to her as Mother Theresa when introducing her to those in my life and to you, Dear Reader, is that her name actually is Theresa.

Valet Golf

So my Vertigo lasted only about two and a half weeks, and I give all the credit for my cure to Dr. Cheryl, my acupuncture/chi-ropractic guide. The combination of massage, acupuncture, and a few neck adjustments cleared up the majority of my vertigo so that I was able to drive a car and function like a normal human being. Thank you Dr. Cheryl.

Prior to that, however, I was totally dependent on others for basic activities, of which there were more than you might think, since there isn't much that will keep me down. I kept up my business throughout my two vertiginous weeks. My mother drove me to all of my business appointments, not to mention medical ones; she would read a book while I fixed a computer or trained someone. What a trooper!

I wasn't going to stop golfing either. It was bad enough I had missed one week of golf when I was hospitalized; I wasn't going to miss another. So the week after I got out of the hospital, I decided I would play golf in my usual Tuesday league. Jeff put my clubs in the trunk and me in the passenger seat, then drove me (my eyes closed to fight off dizziness) up to our town course. There, I met up with my usual golf buddies, Jeanne and Nancy. They couldn't believe I was there. I said, "I need to do this. I am going to practice driving too. I'll drive a golf cart and see if I'm steady enough to drive my car later." As I said that, I staggered into the Pro Shop to pay for my cart and nine holes. Jeanne saw me walk, and she (who always walked the course) said, "It's pretty hot today; I think I'll ride. In fact, Pam, I think I'll drive!" Well, that was the end of my opportunity to practice driving.

So off we went to the first hole. With a very wide stance, I walked up to the tee, squatted, and placed my tee and ball. I announced to my partners that I would not be able to look up after I hit and asked them to please watch where my ball went. I yelled "Hitting" and hit. They watched in some amazement. I staggered back to the golf cart and Jeanne proceeded to drive me to my ball. This went on until we all reached the green. That was more of a challenge. There, I had trouble looking up from my ball to the hole, so my putting was somewhat erratic. Nancy and Jeanne wouldn't let me pick up my ball from the hole or pick up any clubs off the ground for fear that I would fall over.

In the end, I decided this was the way to golf. Have someone drive you to the course, take out your clubs and put them on a cart; have someone else drive you around in the cart; have your team watch where your ball goes, pick the ball out of the hole and scoop up any clubs lying around on the green. Then call your husband to take you home. I'll call it "Valet Golf."

The Huddle

There I was again sitting in the Treatment Center getting my weekly dose of Magnesium when I started to feel tired. That might have been normal for most patients, but not for me. I didn't get tired when receiving an infusion, and I certainly didn't get tired at 11:30 in the morning. As I was driving home, I felt worse. I didn't say anything to my mom, who was with me at my treatment, but when I got home, I called my only client that afternoon and said I needed to postpone. I immediately curled up in bed and started shivering. *This can't be good,* I thought.

Two hours later, after no sleep to speak of, I got up and took my temperature. 101. I remembered that the nurses and doctor had told me that if I ever got a fever, I was to call them immediately. When I did, I was told "You need to come in right away." So I called my designated driver, Mother Theresa, and said, "If you're free, let's go hang out at the hospital again. I have a fever." So off we went back to the same place we had just left a few hours before.

After a couple of hours of being looked at by the doctors and nurses and prodded with a thermometer several times, an escort arrived with a wheelchair to take me to the sixth floor for admission. Wouldn't you know it. When I got up there, they had my private room, #6039, ready for me. This was the same room I'd had for my three-day stay with Vertigo. And Liz, one of my favorite nurses was the one welcoming me with paperwork to be filled out, a fresh pitcher of hospital water, and a big bag of saline. I felt as if I was home again!

But I saw trouble. It was Friday and our club championship was coming up on Monday and Tuesday, so I had to get out of the hospital no later than Sunday night to make it. I couldn't miss another day of golf, I thought, especially the club championship. So I needed a plan.

I called the night nurse and the nurse's aides in for an emergency meeting. When I explained the situation, they told me that Dr. "R" was on rounds that weekend and didn't let anyone go unless they'd been without a fever for forty-eight hours. Well that wasn't going to work because we were already at the forty-eight hour mark and I was sweating bullets from the fever. The night staff said "Good luck" and I took my two Tylenol before going to sleep.

The nurse's shift changed at 7:30 a.m., and I called another meeting. In our huddle I told them the need-to-get-out-of-here story and they all agreed to help me out. Then Dr. "R" came in for rounds. My nurse, Mary, petitioned a very understanding resident as well as Dr. "R," who said, "Well, I usually don't let patients out unless they have been without a fever for 48 hours." Where had I heard that before? She asked me where I was playing golf and I told her. The resident asked what time I was teeing off, thinking I could possibly get out very early Monday morning if all looked good, and Dr. "R" finally said, "Ok, if you don't have a fever for twenty-four hours and your blood work looks good and you agree to become part of the hospital's Golf Tournament Committee to get patients involved next year, then I'll consider letting you go home Sunday afternoon." I wondered how that last part about a committee had gotten in there, but I wasn't going to argue. "Ok," I said.

My fever spiked at 3:00 p.m. Saturday afternoon. "Crap," I said. Now I couldn't have a fever between Saturday night and Sunday at 3:00 p.m. in order for Dr. "R" to even consider letting me go home. I got the night crew together and said, "All right, this is really a critical night. I need to be fever-free from this point on until tomorrow at 3:00 p.m. Are you with me?" One nurse raised her hand and I immediately called on her. She had so much enthusiasm and team spirit. In response to her "I can put cold towels on you" I said "Perfect, and I like your spirit!"

At 3:50 p.m. on Sunday, John, the nurse's aide, came in to take my temperature. I had been Tylenol-free for 20 hours. The moment of truth loomed. All the nurses were anxiously awaiting the reading. "97.8", he said. "Lacko is out of here!" Yes, it was true. I was going home and it took me less than sixty-five seconds to get my Johnny off and my clothes on. My wheelchair escort arrived within five minutes and reported that Mother Theresa was bringing the Rav 4 around. I was home free. On my way out, I asked the nurses if they would put my name on the door for any future visits. Room 6039 was for me!

Top Ten Benefits of Having Ovarian Cancer

On Labor Day weekend, I held my annual golf tournament, a fund-raiser for the American Cancer Society. Now, Cancer had never been the main focus, but here I was, a living testament to the importance of benefiting the ACS. Yes, we raised and donated money for the ACS, but the tournament itself had always been upbeat and fun. How could I be amusing in front of all the players? Then it came to me. Being bald at the time, I was just the right person to do a David Letterman and announce the "Top 10 Benefits of Having Ovarian Cancer." So here is the list I concocted:

10. *Being able to blame the loss of a golf match on having the big "C"*
9. *Winning a golf match because of a blood infusion the prior day*
8. *Spending hundreds of dollars on full body massages without any complaints from your husband*
7. *Time saved each morning with:*
   No blow-drying
   No shaving
   No eyebrow-plucking
6. *Getting homemade meals after each hospital stay (I even lied once about being hospitalized just to get fabulous lasagna.)*
5. *Having a natural bug-repellant*
4. *Saving hundreds of dollars on hair products and bikini waxes*
3. *Being able to wear a baseball cap and look good in it*
2. *Being able to shock my hairdresser's clients by waiting for their busiest day, walking in, taking my hat off, and saying "Look what you did to my hair!"*
1. *Being selected as the year's Chia Pet holiday season promotion*

Chapter Four: After-Effects

Did You Say Reiki or Raking?

A dear friend of mine was taking courses in Yoga, Reiki and other exercise, health, and healing practices. She asked if she could do Reiki on me. After being stabbed by nurses, poked by my acupuncturist, stone-massaged by my massage therapist, and cracked by my chiropractor, I thought, *Why not!*

So she told her instructor about me, and the instructor suggested that she do "Distance Reiki" on me to start. She said she would ask her instructor how to do it, but I was pretty sure it was simply a matter of sending patients to the Camen Islands for one week (all expenses paid of course) and thinking happy thoughts about them while they lay on the beach drinking margaritas all day. Whatever the case, I was hoping we'd start the Distance Reiki soon, as I needed to prepare for the real raking that would happen in the back yard around November!

Distance Reiki—Very Cool

One Saturday, I was painting the trim in my dining room when the telephone rang. It was my friend who was taking the Reiki course. She said she was at school and the class wanted to perform Distance Reiki on me. I guess she had figured out how to do it, and unfortunately it wasn't going to involve any plane rides to the Camen Islands. She asked if I had ten minutes to spare. "Yes, of course."

She instructed me to lie down in a quiet room and wait. After ten minutes she would call me back. So I and my Type A personality climbed the stairs to my bedroom where I lay down wide awake at 3:00 p.m. on a Saturday afternoon. I hadn't done that in 20 years. As I began to relax, my ears started ringing. *Strange*, I thought, *but then lots of people have that sensation every now and then.*

My friend called back several minutes later and asked how I felt. I told her that the only thing I'd noticed was a ringing in my ears. She said, "Isn't that interesting!" and added that she would talk with me later.

The following week I met with a client who happened to be in that same Reiki class and had also performed the Distance Reiki on me. She said that when she'd visualized my head, her hands had started to tingle around my ears. Weird, huh? As you'll remember, the needles for acupuncture wouldn't stay in my ears and not long before the Reiki experiment, I'd had vertigo—an inner ear imbalance.

I wondered if the chemo had gotten stuck up there. I couldn't wait for the "Close up Reiki" session. Maybe my ears would fall off.

Hair and Magnets

My hair was growing back slowly on my head and fast everywhere else. No longer did I have the luxury of extra time in the morning from not needing to shave. I had been watering my head every day for two months, hoping for a good thick crop, but it looked as if it would grow in as thin and straight as it was before. Jeff said I looked like Eddie Munster from the Adams Family with my widow's peak in the front. Oh well, Eddie Munster was better than Yule Brynner or Telly Savalis.

I was still going to the hospital weekly for Magnesium infusions. After three months of infusing, I should have been full of mag, bubbling over with it and so magnetic I'd be sucked into the kitchen and stick to the refrigerator. But no, I was still eating almonds, taking prescription mag daily, and getting a bag of it weekly.

As a precaution, just before going into the kitchen I would slowly peek around the corner and stick my finger in the air toward the fridge. You never know.

Feet, Legs, Torso and All

After my first experience with Distance Reiki, I began three sessions of "Hands On" Reiki. Three wonderful ladies who had met each other at a Reiki course performed the healing ritual on me after my magnesium infusions each week. It had always been extremely difficult for me to relax—even during my hot stone massages I typically yakked up a storm. But *this* relaxed me entirely. The Reiki Masters concentrated in total silence. There was soothing music in the background and candles filled the room with warmth and a pleasant scent.

Each of them worked on a part of my body (one on my feet and legs, another on my torso, and the third on my head). While they rotated positions, all parts of my body were always concentrated on at the same time. To say this was comforting is an understatement! After each session we talked about what I felt and what they felt. Each time they put their hands on my abdomen (approximately where the cancer was) I felt an overwhelming heat in that area, and they said they felt tingling or buzzing in their hands. Interesting.

What I was most worried about was my ears. Thank goodness they stayed put.

CHAPTER FIVE: MY NEW ADVENTURE

Where's Mom When You Need Her

Now on to my new adventure. Because Ovarian Cancer has possible genetic links to Breast Cancer, I was scheduled for a breast MRI, and remembering the last experience, I thought I would get something to cover my eyes while I was in the tiny machine. Sometimes the mind plays tricks and makes you open your eyes when you really shouldn't, not when the ceiling of the MRI tube is three inches from your face. Not a pretty picture. So a friend gave me a room-darkening eye cover, the kind used to sleep during long airplane rides.

Mother Theresa had gone back to Siesta Key, Florida for a few weeks, so Jeff was my designated driver. My doctor had notified the radiology unit ahead of time that I'd be given the injection of contrast through my port by hand, not by the traditional pump. So our first stop was the Treatment Center to get my port accessed for the test. Ten minutes there and I was off to the Imaging Center. As we waited for my turn, I noticed that Jeff was reading the newspaper with his eyes closed and head tipped. *Oh well, he bores easily,* I thought.

Within a few minutes an orderly called me in. We will call him Charlie. He said, "Please go into that room, undress from the waist up, and put on that Johnny." I wished I had known that a breast MRI was done in the nude. I would not have spent half the morning searching for clothing without any metal snaps, zippers or buttons. Anyway, I got undressed, slipped into my Johnny, and came out with my eye cover in hand, at which point Charlie said, "Oh, I'll take that bra for you." This eye cover was about three inches wide and seven inches long. How could he possibly have thought it was a bra? Red flag, red flag.

My port tubing was sticking out of my Johnny, and I explained the situation to Charlie: "We might need some extension tubing for the port, so I brought some along." (Actually, the Treatment Center nurse had given me the tubing). To this, Charlie replied, "Oh we won't be using your port. We will just access a vein." *Oh dear, where is my mother? Where is Jeff? Help, I need help!*

I said, "Listen Charlie, my veins are fried from Chemo. That's why I have a port. No one is going to access a vein here today!" Charlie replied, "I don't want to upset you, Mrs. Lacko. I see some good veins on your hands right here," and he lifted my hand to show me. Little did he know I was going to hit him with that hand if he didn't cut it out. Holding back the urge, I calmly said, "Charlie, I believe you are good at your job and know what you are talking about, but I want you to talk to the Radiologist about this before we go any further." Charlie said, "I will call him when we get you on the table and check with him, but breast MRI results will be compromised if we don't use the appropriate contrast speed through an IV." All I said was "Check with the doctor, please," and off Charlie went.

Another technician came in to get me situated on the table. So I looked down at the table (not really a table but more of a thin slab with a sheet on it) and noticed what appeared to be a pair of ski goggles and two indentations in the sheet farther down the slab. "Interesting," I thought. Then, as the technician explained the position I was to assume, it all became incredibly clear. I was to lie face-down on the slab, putting my mams in the two indentations and my head in the goggles. Meanwhile, Charlie hadn't returned yet. The goggles had a mirror attached so when the user opened her eyes she could see the room and not feel so claustrophobic.

All right, I put away my little bra of an eye cover and proceeded to parachute into place. I didn't have a lot of abdominal strength for getting into the prescribed position, but in the end I did it. Not very gracefully, I might add.

When they put the headphones on, Charlie piped in and said he had spoken with the Radiologist—using the port would be fine. Phew!

Well, Jeff slept through the entire test. When I came out to the waiting room he said, "Where have you been? I've been worried about you!"

My, Aren't We Perky

Good news—the MRI was negative! But with a grandmother who had died of Ovarian Cancer in her mid forties and my diagnosis of Stage II Ovarian at age 47, my oncologist recommended that I get tested for the BRCA1 and BRCA2 mutated gene that would mean my risk of developing Breast Cancer was very high. I knew a bit about this test because my friend Mary Beth had tested positive for the mutation years earlier. One bit of good news: if you have Ovarian Cancer and are related to a sibling, parent or grandparent who had the disease, the blood test is paid for by insurance. Otherwise it would cost $3000 to $4000.

My mother and I filled out thirty pages of family history on both her side and my dad's before I even took the blood test. Two and a half weeks after the test, I got a phone call from the geneticist, who said the results were in. As mom and I sat in the waiting room I placed a bet. I wagered that I wasn't positive for the mutation; mom wagered that I was. I lost the bet.

So walking out of the office I was faced with very scary percentages. I had a 40 percent chance of getting Ovarian Cancer (already been there, done that) and an 85 percent chance of getting Breast Cancer. Ouch. So I took my bald self home, broke the news to Jeff, and two days later, I called my oncologist to say I had decided on a preemptive strike—a bi-lateral mastectomy.

Yup, a double boob job. This would reduce my risk of developing Breast Cancer by over 90%. That was huge, a mathematical no-brainer in my opinion. But just to be sure, I met with all the doctors who would be involved in the procedure and also with the doctors who would manage my overall well-being. They were all on board and concurred with my decision.

The mastectomy would be a lengthy surgery once again and could not take place until my body had fully recovered from the first surgery and six chemo treatments. My red counts were too low, and I continued to receive Magnesium weekly. So until my vitals improved, any surgery was on hold.

While we wait, let's review the options for reconstruction. Option 1 is called a "tram flap." Before I really knew what this was, I was all for it. My perception was that it was a tummy tuck where they extract the fat from your abdominal area and make boobs out of it. Well, I was wrong. Apparently, stomach muscles and fat are attached to a blood supply in the middle of the torso. They actually make an incision from one hip to the other, pull up your fat and muscle, leaving it attached to the blood supply, and put it where your boobs were. Yuk! It would be painful at best and I'd feel tight in my abdominal area forever. Not to mention that parts of my new boobs could die off if the blood supply turned out to be too far away from them.

Option 2 is the implant. With implants, the mastectomy comes first, and while the patient is still on the table, the plastic surgeon puts in these things called expanders. The expanders go under the pectoral muscles and are filled with a little bit of saline. Over the course of the next weeks/months, the plastic surgeon increases the amount of saline in the expanders to get the muscle and tissue expanded to the desired size (if you know what I mean). Then you go back into surgery to get your implants.

Now there are two kinds of implants, Saline and Silicone. Saline implants are like two water balloons on your chest, and yes, they can burst. Initially, I was thinking Saline would be the way to go. If I should be stranded on an island for a long period of time, I would have a water supply. Then I thought about the other things I like to do, including acupuncture. What if my doctor pushed the needle in too far and burst a boob? That might not be covered by insurance. Too dangerous.

The silicone implants got a bad rap several years ago when they were filled with toxic fluid. Now they are built like gummy bears or gelatin. When you cut them, nothing leaks out. They are solid. Most women choose the silicone implants because they don't wrinkle (the saline ones do, when they aren't in their holders, if you know what I mean). So silicone it was.

I asked the plastic surgeon lots of important questions. By the way, he is very good looking and has a wonderful sense of humor. I met with him for about an hour on Halloween. What a treat! One of my questions was "What about my golf game?" He said that during my recovery after the mastectomy, I wouldn't be swinging anything, but that over time I could begin to chip and putt. He said my golf score would actually go down because of the amount of chipping and putting I would be doing. My other question was "How long does it take to complete the reconstruction process?" That's when he said, "When you make a decision to reconstruct, you're married to your surgeon for life." Wow, that was music to my ears. The thought of being married to two wonderful and handsome men really made my day.

He went on to explain that after inserting the implants he would reconstruct everything else with out-patient surgery or in the office, including some tattooing. I'd thought they just glued candy corns to the middle of your implants and maybe used some magic marker to apply the color. He quickly corrected me. I knew right then and there that his name was Doctor Gorgeous.

CHAPTER SIX: My New Jugs

Now that you are prepared for my Mammalian Adventure, I need to complete the tale of the first one. Although my chemotherapy had ended months earlier, I continued to need magnesium infusions weekly. I had been told that this was normal, a side-effect of the Carboplatin (one of the two chemo concoctions) I had been given. So every week I went to the Treatment Center, had my port accessed, and got a magnesium drip.

The weird thing was that although the doctors said my situation was normal, I didn't see any other patients at the Treatment Center getting magnesium infusions. On advice from a friend, I began seeing a naturopath doctor, who immediately thought that I had an absorption issue with minerals. In an effort to improve my red blood counts and my magnesium level, he prescribed several pills and elixirs. So I began taking thirty-one pills a day, not to mention a couple of drops of mushroom extract in my pineapple juice. Well, no go. For all of my daily doses of Gui Pi (pronounced "Gwee Pee" and looking like tiny black ball bearings) and assorted types of magnesium, my counts still remained low.

I finally got frustrated enough to stop one of the oncologists in the hallway while at the hospital. "I'm tired of coming here each week and not making any progress," I said. He suggested I see a kidney specialist, aka Nephrologist. At first I thought he'd said "Neurologist," but thankfully the problem wasn't all in my head.

Soon after, I met Dr. Kaplan and at first was stunned by his introduction. First you need to see him from my perspective. He was a short man, maybe five feet in height, balding, bespectacled, and very happy. Smiling as I offered my hand, he nodded, extended two fingers for a makeshift handshake, and took a seat at his desk. He opened my file and said he had read up on me before I came in. Then he started to stumble with his words: "If you hear hoof horses, I mean hoof beats, I mean horse hoofs in Central Park, then it's not a Zebra." My response was simply "What?" To which he replied, "You know, if you hear horse hoofs in Central Park then it's probably a horse and not a zebra." When I asked what that had to do with me," he answered, "Well, if a Zebra jumped over the fence from the Bronx Zoo and went into Central Park, then it could be a Zebra." I was sitting there on the examining table scratching my head and wondering if I should have gone to the Neurologist instead of this guy.

Dr. Kaplan then explained that my case was clearly Carboplatin-Induced Magnesium Deficiency. *Duh,* I said to myself. He said that we would confirm this with a 24-hour Urine Capture Test and some blood work, all to be done the following week a day prior to my next magnesium infusion. He explained how the test works and left the room for a few minutes, coming back with two half-gallon plastic milk jugs. He handed them to me, said I should use these for my capture, and began to walk me to the check-out desk, at which point I said, "How can I pee into one of these jugs. They won't fit in the toilet!" His response was "Oh yeh, you need a hat." Well, I knew what he meant. Not a hat for my head but a hat for the toilet to catch my urine. When I said "I don't have one, do you?" he walked down the hall, opened a closet door, and came back with a hat. As I stood there with my two milk jugs and "hat," I realized I would have to carry them through the waiting room filled with people and through the rest of the hospital. Everyone would stare into my secret life, and I'd probably be arrested for stealing hospital supplies. So I asked Dr. K. if he had a couple of bags I could use. Back to the closet he went. I waltzed out of the hospital with two large Target bags filled with my jugs and hat! I felt as if I had just done some Christmas shopping at the mall.

Holiday Trimmings

Perhaps my head was indeed affected by chemo: I've become alarmingly non-sequential and now find myself wanting to add a postscript concerning my Bad Hair Days. My first chemotherapy appointment had been on February 29th, 2008. Exactly three weeks later I had lost most of my hair, and the rest I buzz-shaved. I was pretty much bald by April. My last chemo was in June, and my first hair showed up in August. In four and a half months my hair had grown about an inch, maybe a little more on the sides. So I thought it was time. I called Donna the Hairdresser and scheduled an appointment for a trim. I walked in, took off my baseball hat (I'd been wearing a series of these since May), and all in the salon giggled a bit. For me this was a big deal. I was hoping Donna could do wonders with the amount of hair I had grown. It had covered my ears and was long on the back of my neck. Well, ten minutes later, I walked out with a shorter, neater 'do but still required a hat.

I immediately went home and washed my hair with volumizing shampoo, hoping to move things along. I seriously considered using the Chia Pet formula or fertilizer if things didn't improve within the next month.

The Crew

This story is dedicated to the wonderful nurses who work in the Treatment Center. They became an integral part of my recovery process. Among their other tricks was a means of accessing ports when they acted up, and yes, that happened to me a few times.

My port, which is still in operation, was surgically implanted under the skin in my chest, appropriately enough just above my left "jug." It is connected to an artery so that drawing blood and administering meds can be done more easily. Convenient though it is, it can easily be infected, so the nurses need to wear masks and specially treated gloves (not the ivory-colored ones they normally use). And everything has to be sterilized before they access the port. Naturally, I am allergic to the sterilization process and the bandages the nurses use. So for me, the process has to be customized.

Accessing the port doesn't hurt too much, but they do have to push a needle through the skin to get at it. So I numb it up with Lidocaine about two hours before my appointments. It helps a lot.

During the days of my treatments, one of the nurses, Carm, was very animated. She sang while she worked, told jokes and generally kept everyone upbeat. Another of Carm's ways of keeping our minds off our situation was asking TV Trivia questions. One day Carm's question was "What was the little girl's name in *Lost in Space*?" That kept us all busy for awhile, since the rule was that laptops couldn't be used. By the way, it was Angela Cartwright.

The first time a tehnician couldn't get a good blood return out of my port, which meant that the port had not been accessed properly and was not ready to receive meds, Carm came right over. She told me to point my head to the east and lift up my left arm. Then she pushed the reclining chair so far back that I was pretty much upside down. She told me to begin singing the *Star Spangled Banner*. I did, and Carm chimed in as well. Before I knew it, not only was the blood coming out of the port, but everyone in the Treatment Center was standing with their right hands over their hearts, singing *The Star Spangled Banner* with us.

Playing the C Card

Recently, while I was talking with someone just diagnosed with Breast Cancer, we found ourselves joking about "playing the C card." How many times had I done that since I was diagnosed? Not enough. Playing the C card is probably the best gift this disease can give you. Think of all the nonsense you wish you'd never become involved in. Whether it's a book club or an organization from which you want out, now you can say "I have Cancer and I really can't do this anymore." And guess what—everyone understands. They give you an automatic release without an ounce of guilt.

Try to do the same thing without a good excuse like Cancer, and everyone gives you the hairy eyeball. You know, the "how can you do this to us" look. And how many of us would actually leave a book club or organization? We just suck it up each time we're scheduled to go and grit our teeth through it.

Here's an idea: you could always pretend you have the big C. Shave your head, eyebrows and arm hair. Then put on some white makeup and let them know you will no longer participate.

A Free Lunch

Cancer is a strange disease. You don't necessarily feel bad when you have it. At least I didn't. I had no idea that I had a tumor, and although I had symptoms, they weren't classic Cancer symptoms. It's only when you go through chemotherapy that you feel really sick. Some chemo treatments, like the one I had, kill off fast growing cells (Cancer cells and hair-growing cells) so you lose your hair within the first three weeks of your first treatment. Then outwardly it's obvious you have Cancer. No one would ever know otherwise.

So I wore a wig for a period of time, especially when I went out of my house, and then I eventually migrated to baseball caps when it got too hot for the wig. It's pretty obvious that you are a member of the Big C Club when you wear a baseball cap on a bald head, not to mention the lack of eyebrows and eyelashes. So people I didn't even know would ask me how I was. I feel bad for Cancer patients undergoing treatment that doesn't kill their hair cells—no one knows they have the disease, and they don't get the sympathetic notice they deserve.

Here's an example of the royal treatment I received. Jeff and

I went to a local restaurant for lunch one day. I had my Breast Cancer baseball cap on (they haven't made one for Ovarian Cancer—maybe that will be my next endeavor) and when we were ready to leave, the waitress touched my arm and said, "Good luck with everything." Don't get me wrong—it was a nice gesture, but I was thinking she could have said "Good luck with everything, lunch is on me!" Whatever happened to a free lunch? I might design an Ovarian Cancer hat in the shape of an Apricot. Apparently that's the ovary's size and shape, pre-C.

No, I'm Not Dead

There were several months when I was feeling great and getting back to a normal life with my Cancer in remission, and it finally dawned on me that I hadn't posted anything on my Cancer blog for quite awhile. One day I ran into someone I knew who said, "Thank God I ran into you. I haven't seen any new writings on your blog, and I thought you had taken a turn for the worse." Well that was far from the truth, and in fact I was feeling better than ever. I had finally started to frequent the gym again, trying to shed those chemotherapy pounds and get my muscles back up to snuff for golfing. I was hitting the links twice a week and walking the course, which was a huge improvement over where I'd been just two months earlier. All was good.

I didn't want to miss a single joy. In fact, I had to reschedule my next surgery (Preventative Bi-lateral Mastectomy) for a bit later in the summer because I found out that *Earth, Wind and Fire* was coming to town. I really wanted to see them perform. The boobs could wait. The last time I'd been at a concert in town, though, I'd ended up in the hospital with Vertigo, so I was crossing my fingers that I would be able to walk a straight line after this one.

Another thing that kept me busy was completing an article I'd been asked to write for the *International Journal of Healing and Caring*. I used a couple of the stories from my blog and called the article "Prescription: Humor!" The writing, which I did in concert with the journal's very helpful editor, took several weeks and iterations, but it was a fun thing to do and led to the book you hold in your hands.

So I wasn't dead after all, just very busy, moving forward, and looking ahead to Perky Boobs for my birthday!

CHAPTER SEVEN: I NEED TO GET SOMETHING OFF MY CHEST!

It had been almost one year since I had tested positive for the BRAC1 gene mutation, which made me predisposed to develop Breast Cancer, and I'd been given lots of time to prepare for my next surgery. On Thursday, September 17th my good-looking plastic surgeon, Dr. G., would come into the pre-op room, draw lines on my breasts to mark where the incisions should be, and off we 'd go. I hoped that my breast surgeon would be able to cut inside the lines!

I started wondering how much weight I'd lose when they took them off. Two pounds, four, thirty? Wouldn't that be great? So, I thought I would run a little contest on my blog. I called it *Guess How Much My Boobs Weigh.*

When I went in for the pre-op appointment with Dr. Wilson, the breast surgeon, she went through a very thorough description of the surgery and what was to follow. When she finished, she asked my mother and me if we had any questions. I asked, "Can you weigh my breasts after you take them off?" She said, "I've never been asked that before. Why do you want them weighed?" I told her about the blog contest, and after she had finished laughing, she explained that they always weigh the breast tissue anyway, so that wouldn't be a problem.

When I asked her how much she thought they might weigh, she explained that everything medical is weighed in grams. So I instructed my blog readers to send their guesses in grams and even suggested a handy conversion website.

I gave everyone three weeks to send in their guesses and assured them that a prize would be awarded after the surgery.

And the Winner Is...

Over one hundred women and one man participated in this "guess my boob weight" contest. I received guesses on the blog and through e-mail. Some people thought I was kidding and just sent notes telling me that I was funny. I replied with e-mails assuring them that I was serious about my boobs. Before I announce the winner, I want to highlight the methods used by some to guess the weight.

One person actually weighed one of her own boobs on a meat scale in her kitchen, then added or subtracted depending on how she thought I compared. Another weighed a bagel and then a banana (why a banana and not a peach, I'm not sure). And yet another went around the house holding her own and calculating.

I did not give weight much thought, as I was thinking more about the surgery and the reconstruction to follow, so it never dawned on me that one breast might be a different size than the other. Well lo and behold, they were different.

After I shared the contest specifics with my breast surgeon, I told my plastic surgeon about it. He too laughed and thought it was a novel idea. When the surgery was over and he met the family, making sure that Jeff and mom knew all was well, he was especially concerned about registering the exact weight of both breasts. He sat in front of the family and began writing the weights on his scrubs. Then he said, "I'm not sure about the right breast. Wait here, I'll be right back." How about that? My surgeon was all about the contest!

He came back and reported the exact weight, which Jeff logged into our home filing system for my future reference. Now here are the stats: the left breast weighed in at 512 grams and the right at 631 grams . (Yes, I 'd been lopsided all my life). And the grand total: 1143 grams. Do the math. That's two and a half pounds.

We had guesses ranging from .64 grams to 144596.96 grams, and the one that came the closest was 1170.34, sent in by a friend of mine who works out with me at our local gym (she must have peeked in the changing room). Her prize was a $100 gift certificate to Victoria's Secret.

Thanks to all who participated in this wacky contest. I appreciated your support and compliments!

After learning the actual weight, a friend asked, "Did you know that your boobs weighed the same as two frozen bags of peas?" I'd never thought of making that comparison.

Nerves

Because I'd had so many months to mentally prepare for this double mastectomy, I was pretty calm on my ride to the hospital. When I arrived, I filled out my paperwork and took a seat next to all of the other patients in the waiting room. Jeff and Mother Theresa were with me when the nurse came out and called my name. We all got up, and she said, "Oh, just Pam right now." So I went through the big double doors, and the first person I spotted was my plastic surgeon, Dr. Gorgeous. After we exchanged pleasantries, off I went to one of the beds behind curtains.

The nurse handed me a Johnny, a pair of no-skid socks, and a surgical hat to change into. I don't know about you, but I often worry that they don't give you enough time to change, so I rushed to take off all of my clothes and put on the hospital gown and socks. I thought the hat could wait. As I squeezed into the gown, I noticed that the sleeves were a bit tight and uncomfortable. I was thinking that they should really make these gowns a bit larger. It's bad enough you have to wear the things; at least they could make them comfortable.

I changed in record time and sat there on the bed for quite awhile, waiting for someone to come. You know, you wait there in that casual but uncomfortable pose on the bed, trying to look graceful and experienced. However, I did notice that I could barely move my arms. Finally Dr. G. walked in, put his hands on my shoulders and asked, "Are you a little nervous?" "No. Why?" I asked, to which he responded, "Because your arms are not in the sleeves of your hospital gown. You've gotten them in between the snaps on the sleeves. It must be uncomfortable." He gave me a reassuring nod and said he would help me correct the problem after he drew some lines for the surgery.

He then took out a purple marker and started to draw a line from my neck down below my breast line. He said that my right breast was larger than my left, which he would correct by removing a bit more skin on that side. I was fine with that. When I was done, I had a purple road map on my chest. He then helped me by unsnapping the sleeves, which let the blood rush back into my hands and fingers, and snapped me up the correct way. He gave me a big hug and said, "I'll see you after the surgery." I wasn't nervous at all!

The surgery was scheduled for noon. I had arrived, changed, and been made into a piece of purple marker art by 11:00 a.m. I proceeded to wait four more hours with Jeff, Mother Theresa and Pastor Laura before I was wheeled into surgery. A friend/client who was performing surgery that morning came by to wish me well and let me know that my breast surgeon had performed an emergency surgery, which was why mine had been delayed. Thank goodness for him. And thank goodness I wasn't an emergency, not yet at least.

I hadn't had anything to eat or drink since 8:00 p.m. the night before, and it was quite annoying when the anesthesiologist came in to ask Jeff and Mother Theresa if they wanted coffee or soda. The nurse presented them with meal tickets for lunch. I gritted my teeth.

Once in the operating room, I was given something in my port, and I dozed off. Hours later I awoke in the Recovery Room asking for ice chips, water or anything liquid! I noticed at that time that they had placed an IV in my right arm, but I didn't care because they had done it while I was asleep.

My chest was numb, and even a year later, parts of my chest were still numb. That was not expected. I had talked to many women who had undergone this procedure, and no one had mentioned numbness. The mystery was solved when my plastic surgeon explained that all of the nerve endings in my chest had been cut. He said I would feel some tingling and other sensations after a time and that eventually, after a year or more, feeling would return, all of which has occurred. Interesting. I guess nerves did play a big part in this surgery!

Step Away from the Bed

When you are hospitalized, a "blood nurse" (that's what I call them) shows up once a day to take blood so your doctors can keep track of your progress. This person's only job is to go from room to room with her "blood kit" and poke a needle in each patient's arm, drawing the amount of blood specified on the doctor's order form. So the morning after my surgery, in popped the "blood nurse." She set her kit down next to me on the bed and said, "Hi, I'm here to take some blood." I looked at my right arm and saw that I still had my IV from the surgery. This reminded me that it hurt. So I said to the blood nurse, "If you can get blood out of my IV, help yourself. If not, the blood needs to come out of my port and we'll have to get my nurse."

Well, she got all high and mighty and said I had great looking veins in my left hand. I pulled my arm back to my bed and repeated my demand. She looked so annoyed that I pressed my call button. I explained the issue to the voice on the other end, and momentarily my nurse arrived, sending the blood nurse on her merry way to the next room. Phew!

My nurse checked my chart, agreed that all blood should

come out of my port, and even moved my IV to the port once it was accessed. My arm felt better and my nerves felt better too. It would have gotten ugly with that bloody nurse if the other hadn't stepped in.

Wrapping and Ornaments

When I woke up the next morning, I realized I had a room-mate. The curtain was drawn between us and I couldn't see her, but I could hear her. I called over and introduced myself as the flat-chested woman from Simsbury. She said, "My name is Gloria." She apologized for having the curtain drawn, explaining that she needed to use the portable commode and didn't want to gross me out. So we knew each other simply by voice for the next twenty-four hours.

At one point during the afternoon, I heard a large bang on Gloria's side of the curtain. Being in no shape to jump out of bed and see what had happened, I yelled to her. She said that she was itching badly and that her call button (the combo remote for the TV and nurse alarm) had fallen to the floor. Now I realized that I was itching too. It was either the power of suggestion or a reaction to the pain meds. So I told her, "I'll call for some Benedryl for the two of us." I did that, and the Benedryl worked wonders. Needless to say, Gloria and I were buds from that point forward, sight un-seen!

One of the doctors had been in that morning to check on me. He had checked my incisions by simply pulling back my ace bandage (at least that's what the beige covering looked liked) and peeking down at my chest. He also "checked my drains." Now both surgeons had told me that I would have drains and that they would be the worst part of this entire ordeal. I couldn't see them and quite frankly I couldn't feel them. In fact, I couldn't feel a thing. I was numb. Every eight to ten hours, the aide would come in to "empty my drains" and would write on the white board how much fluid she had emptied out of each. There were four drains , two on each side.

That Friday night, I was encouraged to get up and walk around the floor. You know, do laps. So the nurses pinned my drains to my Johnny, put another Johnny over my shoulders to close up my backside, and off I went. Two laps the first time I tried. Hours later, I was up to ten laps. Since the hospital floors was circular, the nurse's station was in the middle, and you passed it while doing your laps. It reminded me of Roller Derby, and I started to get a bit competitive with the other patients. There was an older gentleman across the hall who was walking too. I tried not to knock him down when I lapped him. I almost threw him the elbow, but held back! The nurses were getting nervous by this time and suggested I go back to my room. All right, there was always tomorrow, when Mathew (my son) could bring me my helmet and elbow pads!

The next morning it was looking pretty good for early dismissal. I was up and walking, blowing up the lung-tester device and feeling pretty good. I was told that I would have the drains in for another five to ten days, but I wanted very much to take a shower before I left the hospital. So at 2:00 p.m. Mother Theresa announced to the nurse that I needed to shower before I left and that we needed all hands on deck.

The first thing to explain is how these drains are attached. They consist of IV tubing that goes through your armpit (yup, there is a hole in your armpit for each drain). and they are sutured to the skin under your armpit. The drains hold body fluid, and if they are full they pull on the stitches and skin. Hence, you need something that you can pin the drains to while showering.

Unbelievably, not one nurse or aide could come up with a plan. So I remembered my plastic surgeon telling me that women have used yarn, string or fabric belts, placing them over their necks for pinning the drains. I explained this to the nurses, and one then came back with a short ace bandage. "Perfect!" I said.

So off to the shower I went with my drain-sling and my hospital towels the size of postage stamps. On my way, I saw Gloria (the bathroom was on her side of the room) and told her I was off to shower and go home. She was very pleased but told me that she herself would remain in the hospital at least another day. I hoped Gloria would be ok.

When I took off my Johnny in the bathroom, I looked down to see a very wide beige ace bandage type of thing wrapped around my chest. My mother started to unwind it, discovering that it went on for miles. It had to be 10 feet long.

Although showering was awkward, I prevailed, washing my hair and anything else I could reach, and came out shivering, hoping to be wrapped up and warmed up by my oversized thick bath towel at home. Unfortunately, I awoke from that fantasy when I was patted down with those postage stamp, thin white hand towels. Hypothermia was setting in by the time I was able to dress.

First we had to put that bandage back on. It took me, my mother, and one nurse ten minutes to wrap that thing around me. It felt like an eternity. Mom was on one side of me and she would do her side, then pass the bunch of bandage over to the nurse, who would do her side. Then back to mom. It was like putting lights on a Christmas tree. Guess where the drains went. We pinned them to the bandage. Ornaments on a tree! It was finally time to go home. I wondered how long I would need to wear the bandage.

The Look of In-de-cision

When a woman has a mastectomy, one or a double, all of the breast tissue must be removed, including the "candy corns," as I referred to them in my first meeting with my plastic surgeon. To do this, the breast surgeon cuts a circular incision and removes everything in there. The skin stays but that's about it. When I think about it, it's like carving a pumpkin from the top and scooping out all of the insides.

After the breast surgeon gets done removing tissue, the plastic surgeon comes in and puts the expanders in under the "pec" muscles, fills them up with some saline, then sews or glues the two flaps of skin together (upper and lower) on each breast. So my scar looks like the face of indecision. It's neither a smile nor a frown. And with the scar from my hysterectomy, I'm on my way to having a very creative art project on my torso.

Fill Her Up

Let me start by saying that my plastic surgeon is a very happily married man with children. Too bad. He is a very handsome man with a fabulous personality. He is funny, empathetic, caring and most of all makes you feel that you are the only patient he has. I cannot say enough about him.

At my first post-operative appointment, I learned that 250 cc's of saline had been put in my expanders during the operation. Dr. G's Physician's Assistant, Meghan, told me that they usually fill the expanders with 50 to 100 cc's of saline. She said that the surgery had gone so well that they'd put in more than usual. That's why I had cleavage after the surgery. When I looked in the mirror, I thought they hadn't taken everything. I still had little bumps. Apparently that was the saline in the expanders. So essentially I started with a small A cup. That just meant it would take less time to get to my desired size, whatever that might be.

Three weeks out of surgery, I was scheduled for a "fill up." I didn't really know what to expect, but after what I had been through, this couldn't be that bad. The object of a "fill up" is to inject 60 cc's of saline in each expander (fake boob) every ten to fourteen days. They start by using a "port finder" that locates the metal ports under the skin. Then they put a needle in each port to shoot in the saline. I must admit I started to get nervous as soon as I changed into my Johnny. I began to think I should invest in my own Johnny so I could get the right size! My first question was "Does the needle hurt?" Both Dr. G. and his assistant Meghan said that they had performed this procedure on hundreds of women and maybe one had felt pain. Still, I decided that I would play it safe for the next fill up and use my numbing cream beforehand, as I did for my other port when I went in for blood tests. I was determined to be doubly numb. Better safe than sorry. I wondered if I would have to specify regular or premium for my fill up.

A Fill Up and a Leak

I should tell you that the expanders are not round. So when I stood in front of the mirror, it looked as if I had two of those new Thomas' square bagels I've seen in the bread section of the supermarket. At least the permanent implants would be round, more like a true Thomas's bagel, without the hole of course.

The fill up process started with a nurse and a "port finder," a small plastic device with a magnet in the center of it. The nurse moved it around each square bagel until the magnet pointed straight down. Then she took a purple marker, outlined all sides of the device, connected the dots, and drew an X on each of my bagels. The center of each X marked the center of the port beneath.

Next, Meghan came in to administer the saline injection. She warned, "You might not want to watch this the first time," as she took out an enormous syringe the size of Montana and filled it with the saline. Then she added a six-inch needle to the end and approached the examining table. Because I was in a Johnny (yes one of those again), I couldn't run. Heeding Meghan's advice, I closed my eyes tight, gritted my teeth, and waited for the pain. No pain. There was a little pressure, but no pain. Then I realized why—my chest was numb from so much nerve-cutting. Thank goodness for that!

After the first fill up, I sported a modest B cup bust from the 310 cc of saline in my expanders, but unfortunately they were still square. I couldn't wait for my new round ones!

That same afternoon, Jeff and I started draining our waterbed (it had sprung a very slow leak) so we could change out the mattress. Jeff went off to Cape Cod in the afternoon with Mathew for a soccer tournament, and at some point in the evening the bed stopped draining (although there was still quite a bit of water left in the mattress). So I took the hose out of the bed and left with my daughter for a college tour in Boston.

Well, I'm sure you can tell what came next. When we got home there was water coming through my son's bedroom ceiling, and our bedroom above his was completely flooded. Here I was with my mother, daughter and two golden retrievers, knowing we couldn't do a darn thing about it. So I called in the troops. Our neighbors and Becca's strong guy friends came to our rescue. Although it took eight of them, they cut the mattress, bailed the water out of our bedroom window, and eventually threw the mattress out of the window too. What a mess, but they were great and cleaned up every bit of water with towels and sponges. So although I got filled up that weekend, I leaked a bit too! I hoped it wasn't an omen.

And one other thing: I started sloshing. Yes, sloshing. I swear I could feel the saline moving around in my expanders. I even asked someone if they could hear the sloshing as I moved my torso around and around. They said no, but I could swear I heard and felt sloshing. I would ask Dr. G. about it when I went for my next fill up.

Wireless

While I was in Victoria's Secret with my daughter about midway through my reconstruction process (who is Victoria by the way?), she was asked if she wanted to be fitted for a bra. Of course she said yes, and they proceeded to show her the most expensive bras in the store. In the meantime, I was wandering about looking casual. I was the only other person in the store. One of the two salespersons came up to me and asked, "Would you like to be fitted too?" Instead of saying "I'm all set," I blurted out "I recently had a double mastectomy" (like she really wanted to know) "and

I won't need a bra for the next few months." Casually she offered me a looksie at the type of bra I would need after my implants were "installed." The wireless bra is apparently the bra of choice for women with implants. I chuckled because of the irony—as a computer consultant, I'd thought I was already wireless!

Topping Them Off

On December 15, 2009, my expanders were topped off with an extra dose of saline to further stretch my "pec" muscles for the implant surgery. I'd started with 250 cc's of saline on Sept. 17, 2009 and had worked my way up to 610 cc's in each. I was fine at 550 cc's but needed one more injection to give my surgeon a little room to work. I was sloshing more than ever now, and the expanders had moved a bit under my armpit, causing the swaying of my arms to sound a lot like thighs rubbing against corduroys. Whenever I heard the sound, I would look behind myself for whoever was making it. Needless to say, I was anxious for the next surgery, which was scheduled for Thursday, January 28, 2010. New boobs for the New Year!

I spoke with my plastic surgeon about what to expect at my last fill up. Here is what he explained. Silicone implants are extremely expensive, and not every woman will have the same size implant on each side. So essentially Dr. G. had ordered three implants for each side; a size smaller, the exact size I wanted, and a size larger. In addition, he would have three "sizers" for each side. These were preliminary prototypes to show how the final implants would look.

They would put me to sleep, he said, then open up my masectomy incisions, take the saline out of my expanders, remove the expanders, put in the sizers, sit me up (while I was out like a light bulb), and check it all out, adjusting the sizers as necessary. This would have to look pretty weird. There I would be, anesthetized, unable to hold my stomach in or my head up, while they checked out my new boobs. I would probably drool as well. And the whole crew in the operating room would be in on this. I thought it was pretty interesting, so I asked Dr. G. if he would take pictures. He said no. Bummer.

Anyway, if it looked as if my left side needed a larger size than my right, he would put the appropriate sizers in for a visual. When he determined what size should go where, he would replace the sizers with the real implants, using only two of the six in the end.

No Bells or Whistles

After the double mastectomy, I was given a laminated card with the picture of an expander on the front and serial numbers on the back. Looking closely at the picture, I would have thought I was looking at a thick jelly fish that had eaten a large black coin. The shape wasn't round, but more oval. The color was gray and it was obviously "expanded."

I was told that this was my ID card in case I needed to take a plane somewhere or walk into a courtroom. Apparently the ports in these expanders are made of metal and will set off any metal detectors. I was also told not to have an MRI while they were in me. It hurt just thinking about that.

I carry this ID card proudly in my wallet right next to the ID card for the port that is still in my chest, although that one is plastic and not metal. I've shown my expander ID card to a few of my friends, and although they don't seem impressed, I feel pretty darn important.

When I was traveling to Florida in January of 2010 for a week's vacation at my mom's (just before my surgery), I was told that I would need to show my ID when going through the metal detector at airport security. I was excited to say the least, until I read about that underwear bomber incident on Christmas Day. Surely security would be stepped up by the time mom and I flew on New Year's Day. I got to thinking that getting patted down by a female TSA agent would not be any fun and could delay our trip at the very least.

Along with reminding me to bring my pills in my carry-on bag, mom made sure I had both my driver's license and my Boob ID Card (BIC) on hand when we arrived at the airport. Our first stop was checking bags and getting our boarding passes. I handed my license and BIC to the baggage handler, who either didn't bother noticing that I'd handed him two forms of ID or wasn't impressed by the picture of the jelly fish who had eaten a black coin. He stuffed both cards back in my hand and told me to proceed to the airport security line with everyone else.

In line, I was getting anxious about approaching the agent who checks IDs along with tickets. When I gave her both IDs she looked at me, creased her eyebrows, and handed everything back, telling me to move forward to the x-ray conveyor belt. At this point I was feeling less than important, in fact downright ignored.

You see, I had envisioned that a TSA agent would escort me to a special room or section of the airport and do the "wand thing," manually scanning my body for metals. So far no special attention had been given to me or mom, and at this point I was removing my shoes, jacket and laptop, placing them on the x-ray belt for scanning. Now I was thinking my big moment would happen when I walked through the metal detector. They would tell me to "step to the side, ma'm," and everyone in the airport would be a witness to the ensuing wand-scan. My condition would be obvious to everyone when the TSA agent made circular motions in the air in front of my "breasts," causing a high-pitched ringing as the wand passed over the metal ports. I slowly walked toward the metal detector with my ID extended to the agent on the other side. He watched as I walked through the detector and gave me a nod, indicating that everything was fine.

The alarm didn't go off at all. The detector didn't detect my metal ports. I was so disappointed. No one cared about my BIC, and there were no bells or whistles as promised. It was a real let-down.

As we boarded the plane, I was starting to think about all of the other metal things that people might have on them or in them that didn't get detected. Better yet, I told myself, let's not think about that.

Can I Try Yours?

As I sat at home on the eve of my boob implant surgery, I laughed out loud, thinking of a situation I'd encountered just a few days earlier. First, a little background. Soon after my surgery, I was contacted by a woman in town; let's call her Julie. She knew about my Cancer journey (it had been widely reported, not least of all by the 5 o'clock news) and wanted advice. She explained that she had been diagnosed with Breast Cancer and had decided to have a double mastectomy followed by reconstruction. I learned that although she was unsure about any post-surgery treatment she might face, she was very firm in her decision.

We talked over the phone a few times about the surgery, the drains, and the tricks I had learned to cope with the discomfort of the mastectomy and reconstruction. After a few weeks she called to ask if she could drop off a book for me to read (*Cancer Vixen,* a memoir written in comic strip form). I said sure. When the doorbell rang, I came face to face with Julie for the first time. She was a very petite and pretty woman of about fifty-five or sixty, although she looked much younger. Her chest (for some reason that's where my eyes always went after my surgery) was a small size A and very suitable for her frame. She explained that she was recovering nicely from her surgery and that the small bumps on her chest were the beginnings of reconstruction. I thought she would have a couple of fill-ups and be done with the whole thing.

I went through the holidays focusing on my own health and fill-ups, then went to Florida for my mini-vacation to see Mother Theresa. When I got home, I realized that I hadn't returned Julie's book, so I stopped by her house one day out of the blue. She lived in a very populated neighborhood at the end of a cul de sac. I walked to the front porch, which was several steps up from ground level (perfect viewing for the neighbors) and rang the doorbell. When she opened her storm door and walked onto the stoop, I couldn't believe the size and shape of her "torpedoes." She looked great! I said, "Whoa, why do yours look so good? Actually, why do yours pop outward? Mine go to the side under my armpits." As I said this, I moved my jacket out of the way and put my hands on either side of my boobs, pushing them inward. "You see, mine go out to the side. They don't look like boobs at all." To this, Julie answered, "Why do yours move? Mine don't move at all. They're hard as rocks."

So as if we were best of friends, we both tried out each other's boobs. She pushed my loose-fitting pair while I tried to budge hers. Unable to believe how hard her expanders were, I asked what the heck they were filling them up with, and she assured me it was saline. She said she had trouble sleeping at night, couldn't really roll over you know, and I could see why. She was at least a D cup at the time I saw her, and she said her doctor was expecting to add two more fill-ups before her implants would be put in. I advised her to stop the fill-ups immediately, worried that she would pop if they added any more to an already full boat.

As I drove away hoping she wouldn't pop, I realized that Julie and I had been on her front stoop fondling each other's breasts without even blinking. And it had only been our second date. Most surprising of all was that we had done our fondling in full view of the neighbors!

A Little Less Droopy

About a week after the implant surgery, I was starting to feel a bit better each day. The surgery had been a success and actually quite quick in terms of hours on the table, but of course I minimized the recovery time I'd need. Here's how it played out.

I couldn't eat anything after 12:00 midnight the night before the procedure, so Jeff and I went out to dinner to "chow down/load up" for the big event. The next day I went to the hospital at 11:30 a.m., scheduled for a 1:00 p.m. surgery. I had a corner pre-op room with one chair, my temporary bed, and several attentive nurses. A few looked familiar from my surgery in September. They each congratulated me when they found out I was in for the "boob implant surgery" and said my plastic surgeon was the best. I already knew that. It was Dr. Gorgeous' last day of surgery at this hospital, so the nurses and staff had brought in a "boob cake." How did I know? He walked by my pre-op room saying "Save me a boob for later, I have to go into my next surgery." What a guy! I don't like sweets, but that cake was sounding really good right about then.

We had our usual discussion with each nurse who arrived, telling her or him that s/he needed to access my port and start the meds there. Once I was asleep they could try to access a vein in my arm all they wanted to. When they asked if I preferred one arm over the other, I said stay away from my left. They put a long piece of surgical tape on it that said DO NOT USE. I wanted to add DO NOT AMPUTATE EITHER, but they assured me it wasn't necessary.

When Dr. G. came in to talk to me, he took out his infamous purple magic marker and drew lines and circles, which to him meant something important but to me looked like a crude map of Hartford. He said that my right boob was drooping lower than my left and he would have to push it up for the sake of symmetry. He also said he needed to "take in" the one on the left so it wouldn't go under my armpit as the expander had. He gave me a hug and said he would see me in the operating room.

As I waited for Craig, my nurse, to wheel me away, I got to thinking about my drooping right boob. I wondered if that's why most of my golf shots sliced to the right, why my right hip hurt more than my left in exercise class, why I heard better with my left ear, and why I swam in circles. Oh, never mind. Anyway, now I am symmetrical though still square-bageled.

The swelling and fluid, which would subside in time, made my jugs look wider than normal, much like the expanders, but others who had traveled this route said my boobs were perfectly normal and would come into their own very soon. Until then, however, I'd still have square bagels. I wanted mine to look like Julie's!

Showering: A New Olympic Sport

Before surgery, my plastic surgeon had told me that I would be very sore under my right breast and on the left side of my left breast after the surgery. I figured I would get through it with a little pain killer here or there. Was I wrong! When the anesthesia wore off, I was in "take-your-breath-away" pain, mostly from the work done on my right side. I might have had a pinched nerve under the bottom curve of my right breast. I was swaddled in bandaging from the hospital, which was actually quite stylish, and couldn't see where the incisions were, but a major one seemed to be under my right breast.

Driving home, I was just happy to be out of the hospital and was looking forward to my own comfortable bed. I knew I would have to sleep sitting up, just as I'd had to after the last surgery, but I was getting pretty good at it and wasn't concerned. Jeff filled my prescriptions and I took my pain killers every four hours on the dot. When I moved or flexed my pec muscles (by accident) that's when I felt the pain.

Two days after my surgery I wanted and needed to take a shower. It meant not only cleaning up and feeling refreshed but also having an opportunity to take a look at Dr. G's handiwork.

Jeff helped me undo my corset/bandage, which was lavender in color and had ribbing with lace around the edges (this must have been a Victoria's Secret bandage or something). When all the white packing fell to the floor, I was left with my square swollen boobs tattooed by purple marker everywhere. I asked Jeff to see if there was an incision under my right boob. "Nope," he said. Nothing but marker there. So we deduced that the work Dr. G had done to pull that side up must all be internal. Gravity was now my enemy. Without the corset on, my new boob was sagging and the pain was outrageous.

I quickly slipped my right arm under my right breast to relieve the painful pressure on my internal sutures. Then off to the shower. The goal here was to wash with one hand as quickly and efficiently as possible so I could get back into my athletic bra, which would provide much-needed support. The athletic bra was a best friend and a vital part of my support system.

Each day after that I took off my athletic bra, slipped an arm under my boob, washed up single-handedly, and dried off quickly, anxious to slip back into my friendly support system. I got down to 4 minutes, 27 seconds. I've contacted the Olympic Committee and am waiting to learn if this will be a winter or summer sport.

Postscript: I began to wonder if Napoleon Bonaparte had undergone some breast work, which would explain why his arm was always in his shirt. You never know.

Can You Hear That?

The saline in the expanders that I had lived with for three months had a predictable habit. It sloshed! Although I was apparently the only one who could sense the sloshing, it was still very real. Now that my implants were in place, however, the sloshing would be no more.

One morning shortly after the implant surgery, I felt what I took to be heartburn and I pressed my fingers on my chest (there was still very little feeling there). What was that? I heard a mysterious gurgling. It felt weird too. There was no liquid in my new silicone implants, so what was that gurling noise?

I pushed again and heard it once more. A *loud* gurgling. I asked Jeff and my sister-in-law Tracy to listen, and they practically jumped out of their skin. Tracy exclaimed "What *is* that?" I said I didn't know but did know I hadn't experienced it before with the expanders. All that day and the next, I showed off this new trick to anyone at the house. My kids thought I was nuts (nothing new there). The gurgling moved too. The next day it wasn't in the same place when I pressed on my chest.

Turns out there were air bubbles in my chest from the surgery. Those who have had abdominal surgery don't experience this gurgling, since their air bubbles turn into gas and escape through the normal route (the back door). But chest air bubbles have no place to go. I hadn't burped up any, and it had been six days. I made a note to ask Dr. G. about this one at my follow-up appointment. Who would have guessed!

Tootsie Rolls and Erasers

After two post-operative visits with my plastic surgeon, it was time to talk about the next and hopefully final round of reconstruction. When I got the implants in January, Dr. G used a size 600 on the left and a 550 on the right because at the time they looked symmetrical for my body. Well, when the swelling went down and most of the incisions had healed, it seemed that I would look better with a 600 on the right, plus some nip-and-tucking around both to lift and push in. As a result, the next surgery was scheduled for May 20th. Dr. G and I looked at my "before pictures" as he pointed out that my right boob had always been a "low rider." Yes, it had always hung lower than my left, so he could only do so much with what God had given me for a frame. Part of the next surgery would involve nipping and tucking in different areas of my breasts in an effort to make both look as even-keeled as possible. I had always wondered why I leaned to the right all of the time. I thought it was just because I was right-handed!

Then we talked about tootsie rolls and erasers. Yup, you guessed it. It was time for the nipple construction. Depending upon how much skin remains from a mastectomy (and in my case I had all of it), the surgeon can actually use part of it to construct the nipple. This surgery is optional, and at first I thought I wouldn't pursue it, but because we needed to swap out an implant and do some more adjusting, it would be convenient to do it all at once while I was asleep! So here's how the surgery was explained. He would cut a star-shaped incision at the center of each boob, above my existing scar (the one of "in-de-cision"). He would then twist that tissue/skin and sew around it, making what would look like two Tootsie Rolls. They would stick out a good inch for the first couple of weeks, then shrink down to eraser size when the swelling subsided. And I had assumed they just glued on candy corns! What was I thinking?

Over the Hump(s)

February 7, 2010 marked a huge milestone for me and my family. It had been exactly two years since my Ovarian Cancer diagnosis and surgery. Since then I had experienced four surgeries, six chemotherapy treatments, five blood transfusions, over one hundred blood tests, and at least fifteen shots of Procrit. I'd also had two ports, two expanders and two implants inserted, two expanders removed, one wig and two front-zipping athletic bras, one buzz cut, eight haircuts, thirty plus homemade meals from friends, hundreds of get-well cards and e-mails including those from two church school classes and a church in town. I'd attended one support group (Bernie Siegel's), organized two golf tournaments (fund raisers for the American Cancer Society), played thirty plus rounds of golf, worked out a bit at the gym, attended one graduation bald and one wedding without my boobs. In addition, I had joined a bell choir at church, taught drum lessons to local kids, and maintained my computer business. All of which I just loved. I'm exhausted just writing this. At this point, I face no more surgeries. Believe it or not, the last one was the toughest of all of them.

Recovery from it was the most painful, but maybe that's because it was breast augmentation—no pain, no gain. Jeff was just thrilled that the doctors were putting stuff in versus taking it out.

Anyway, my Cancer has been in remission for more than three years. You can never really say you are Cancer-free, but you can say it's in remission. And I know that if it does come back one day, I have learned enough to put it back in its place! We are over the hump or should I say "humps"!

TIPS

1. Get an Advocate. Pick a health advocate from your family or friends. As soon as you have symptoms, confide in someone you trust and someone who can and will speak on your behalf. Make sure this person has access to your health information. You may need to have her/him sign HIPA (Health Information Privacy Act of 1999) release forms for each doctor you visit.

2. Act Now. Never second-guess your gut instinct. I had a friend who had a lumpectomy followed by weeks of radiation and was told by her oncologist that her treatment was complete and that she would be seen again in six months. Two months after treatment, she felt a lump in her other breast and was telling me about it. She said she would have it checked at her six- month appointment. I said, "Wrong! Get off the phone with me, call your breast surgeon's office, say what you have found, and insist that it be checked immediately." She had her appointment two days later, and luckily the problem was only a cyst, but her doctor applauded her for calling immediately. Prompt action against an aggressive form of Cancer can mean the difference between life and death.

3. Information Ownership. Obtain copies of your surgery reports showing how the surgeon performed the surgery, what was found by the pathologist, and the final diagnosis. Also obtain copies of any Ultrasound, MRI, X-ray and biopsy results. If you can obtain and hold onto any visual results of the latter, that would be recommended. You never know when you may need all of this, possibly years down the road. Doctors come and go, and records can get misplaced. Having copies of everything insures that you have control over your health information if you need access to it. This information will also be helpful for your descendants. In my case, I carry a genetic mutation that was likely the cause of my Ovarian Cancer. This genetic mutation may continue in my family, and my medical history will be invaluable to my descendant's physicians.

4. Family Meeting. Everyone in your family and even close friends will have their own questions and concerns about your health and any treatment you may be getting. It is much easier to collectively come up with the questions for a doctor than to bring everyone to an appointment. So periodically (at critical points in your diagnosis and treatment), assemble those close to you, including your spouse, children (depending on age), siblings, parents, and close friends. Then brainstorm, raising all questions and concerns, being careful to document each in writing to take to your next appointment.

5. Never Go It Alone. Always bring someone to each appointment, whether it's a routine check up with the oncologist, a follow-up appointment with your surgeon, or a chemotherapy or radiation treatment. You never know what will be said that you will miss, or what complications might arise from your treatment. If you are going to a key appointment with your doctor to talk about results or future treatment, bring two advocates. One can listen, one can take detailed notes, and the patient can react.

6. Monitor Your Own Stats. Be sure to get copies of your blood work each time you have your blood tested. Ask questions or research each area tested to understand what it is, why it's important if it is not normal, what causes it to be higher or lower than normal, what you can do to help keep it normal, and what to expect during each phase of treatment for your disease. In conjunction with your doctors, investigate supplements and dietary changes that may improve your blood results.

7. Tax Break. Medical bills certainly pile up with a catastrophic illness such as Cancer, so you want to keep detailed records of your out-of-pocket expenditures related to you, your spouse and any dependants you claim in a given tax year. Refer to the IRS website to learn about the specific expenses that can be deducted, begin recording those, and include them in your federal tax return. See http://www.irs.gov/taxtopics/tc502.html. As of 2011, you may deduct only the amount by which your total medical care expenses for the year exceed 7.5% of your adjusted gross income.

8. Be Prepared and Well Informed. Information is power. The more you know about your diagnosis, your treatment and your prognosis, the better off you will be. Seek out other people who have gone through what you are about to go through and learn from their experiences. Ask them what they felt like, what they took for supplements and ate during their treatment. Ask them what made them feel better, what made them feel worse. The nurses in your treatment center will also be invaluable in answering questions about your treatment and reaction to treatments. They see the effects of treatment all of the time and can help you prepare for it.

9. Ask Questions. Each doctor is different. They will provide you with the amount of information they feel they need to. Don't be afraid to ask questions. Many times patients feel that they are taking their doctors away from more important duties by asking questions. Look at a doctor as your answer-center. If you can prepare your questions ahead of time, the doctor will be more likely to answer them.

10. Surgical Scars. Find out what your body will look like after your surgery. Before my double mastectomy my plastic surgeon showed me pictures of what my chest would look like immediately after the surgery. I was shocked, but I had time to prepare myself for the first time I looked in the mirror after my surgery. It wasn't shocking at all. If your doctor doesn't have pictures to show you, research the surgery on the Internet. Also, ask your doctor what you can do to minimize scarring (Vitamin E, Bacitracin, etc.).

11. Drains after a Mastectomy. Most women who have a mastectomy will have drains for a period of time. The drains are annoying, painful, and get in the way of bathing and wearing clothes. Have on hand an ace bandage, fabric belt, or light scarf that you can hang around your neck so you can pin the drains to it to take the pressure off your armpits. Sleeping, bathing/showering, and dressing will be much more convenient.

12. Drain Removal. The removal of the drains is both painful and relieving. Neither numbing cream nor Novocain injection is feasible for the removal of a drain. Just a snip of the suture, a strong pull of the "hose," and out it comes. I had four drains, two in each armpit. I found the longer a drain stayed in, the more annoying it became and the more painful it was to remove. So before my last removal appointment, I took a painkiller to take the edge off. It still hurt but not as much. Talk to your doctor about what you can or if you can take something prior to your drain-removal appointment.

13. Supplements. For me, Vitamin B6 and Glutamine were suggested by the oncology nurse to help ward off neuropathy, a common side effect of my type of Chemotherapy. Talking with other Ovarian Cancer patients who had received the same Chemotherapy treatment, I learned that they were unaware of these supplements. Not every doctor or hospital will advocate supplements, so be sure to ask if there are things you can do to minimize the side-effects (some temporary and some permanent) of your treatment. Personally, I need magnesium supplements because of a permanent magnesium deficiency from my Carboplatin treatment, a deficiency that could not have been predicted or prevented.

14. Accept Help. Your family, friends and neighbors will want to help you in many different ways. Let them! If they want to prepare and drop off meals for you or your family, let them. If they want to take you to a chemo treatment to keep you company and pass the time, let them—if you feel comfortable. If they want to transport your kids or take out the dog when you're at the hospital, let them. People feel better when they feel that they are helping. It makes them feel a part of the process and close to you. Let them help! If you push people away enough times, they may not offer again, especially when you need it.

15. Be Nice to Your Nurses. Unless you have a reason to dislike your nurses, remember that they are there to help you, not to hurt you intentionally. If you are nice to them and understand what they have to do (in particular accessing veins and administering your chemotherapy), you will get the same in return. These men and women leave their own personal lives at the door to try and save yours. They are seldom thanked for what they do everyday and more often criticized and yelled at for simply doing their jobs. Try to be a good patient.

16. Be Open-Minded. Be open-minded about trying different methods of relieving the pain or discomfort related to chemotherapy. I hate needles, so when a friend suggested acupuncture, my reaction was immediately negative. But I tried it and after four or five bi-weekly treatments, I felt relief from the flu-like aches and pains my chemotherapy caused. And when I was stricken with severe Vertigo, so severe that I couldn't walk by myself for two weeks, I turned to acupuncture. The practitioner recognized that I had a large lump on the back of my neck and believed it was toxic build up from the chemotherapy, so she began an intense massage of the area, then did a chiropractic adjustment of my neck (another sort of treatment I might have resisted on other occasions). Within two days I was able to function on my own and drive a car. Now I am much more open-minded when it comes to non-prescription methods of healing.

17. Get Pampered. In addition to acupuncture, I sought out a

Therapeutic Medical Massage professional and began receiving hot stone massages on the fourth day after each of my treatments (that being the worst day for my flu-like aches). This hour-to-an-hour-and-a-half session was not only soothing but gave me the opportunity to relax and focus on my body (not something a type A personality like me could do on my own). My aches subsided for two to three days after each session, enough for me to feel relaxed and build up my strength for the next chemo treatment. I still get a hot stone massage monthly. In addition, I received Reiki treatments, which also allowed me to relax and focus.

18. Don't Sit Around. For me, the aches and pains I experienced for up to five days after each chemo treatment were worse when I sat around thinking about them. I swear I could feel the pinging of the chemo in various parts of my body, and I knew I'd go crazy if I sat still too long. So I decided to do something. I took walks with friends, I worked, I shopped, I golfed (not well), I went to my kids' soccer games and swim meets, and I went out to lunch with friends. I kept busy and tried to keep my mind off of my body. The time between treatments went faster, and thanks to the massage, acupuncture, walks, and golfing, I didn't have time to focus on any discomfort.

19. Surround Yourself with Friends. I never went to a treatment alone. I invited people who offered to take me to do just that. My chemo treatments lasted between six and eight hours, so I usually had someone take me and stay a couple of hours before being relieved by another friend who came for lunch. Finally, another came to spend the rest of the time with me and take me home. This made the time pass quickly. I know that not being alone helped me stay positive.

20. Your Cancer Can Be in Some Ways a Blessing. It is hard to stay positive when you're faced with a deadly disease like Cancer, but if you remain as positive as you can and surround yourself with positive people, you will benefit in the end. Face it: there is nothing you can do to change your diagnosis. My Cancer made me slow down and really focus on myself, my family and those around me. I met so many new and caring individuals, some of them members of my medical staff and some of them other Cancer patients. I also was reminded of who my friends are. So many people offered their support, prayers and time that I was overwhelmed with emotion. I really feel that this time of my life was as much a blessing as it was a challenge.

21. Be Proactive. One way to be proactive is to get your wig before you lose your hair. Don't wait. In fact, once you know that you will lose your hair, make a day of it (not the hair loss but the "wigging"). Go to the Wig Shop with some of your closest friends and have them help you select a style—a new hairdo or a facsimile of the old one. And have fun! Before you lose your hair, get your wig styled by your hairdresser (a wig will need to be cut and shaped before you can wear it out of the box).

22. Tools. Coming out of surgery from my double mastectomy, I had incisions that went from one side of each now-missing boob to the other side. The incisions were about six to seven inches in length. So when I got home and bathed, I needed to find something to put between me and my athletic bra. I used feminine panty liners, which were the perfect length, were sterile, and had an adhesive back so they would stay in place, clinging to the bra. Perfect—much more economical and convenient than costly sterile pads. Moral: be creative and make your own tools that will aid in your recovery.

23. Document Your Medications. If you use a computer or have a family member or friend who does, create a document listing all of your medications, their dosage, frequency, and time of administration. Have copies of this with you always. Every doctor's office will applaud you for having this level of detailed information in such an organized fashion, and you won't have to remember what you take for meds when they ask you—and they will ask you often. It will also be good to have in case an accident or serious medical condition makes you unable to speak.

24. Communicate. It isn't in my nature to talk about my innermost thoughts, especially concerning Cancer, but I do think it was most helpful to me to let all of my friends and family know how I was doing. I chose to do this in part with e-mails. This cut down on the number of phone calls we would have received at the house and allowed people to check in on me at their convenience. In my communications I was very graphic about my diagnosis, treatment, surgeries, etc., which helped everyone know what I was experiencing. But more importantly, I was keeping in touch with the outside world. There were many, many people out there who cared about me and wanted to know how I was doing. And the same will be true for others in my position. So communicate or have someone do it for you so that those who care about you can be part of your healing process.

25. Journal. Another way of communicating I developed (and probably the best thing I could have done) was my creation of a blog on the Internet. I was surprised to find that this was easy to do—and free. There were far more people who wanted to know how I was doing than I could call or e-mail constantly, so a blog was the perfect answer. My intention was to write about the status of my treatment weekly. This became very therapeutic (although I didn't realize it until months later). My blog eventually helped me develop the wacky perspective on my experiences to which you, Dear Reader, have been privy. Those of you facing Cancer or similar medical crises don't have to start a blog, but I would certainly recommend writing things down on paper or on a computer. There can be no better way to get your feelings out, whatever they are.

A Thank You

On my first day
Of treatment called "care"
My body was all nerves—
I didn't know how I'd fare.

The staff was all bustling
Getting needles and kits.
I sat there just staring,
Thinking "This is the pits."

It was my turn next and
A tall nurse approached.
My heart beat faster
As a subject she broached:

"I'm sorry you have cancer.
This must be quite a scare.
But we are here to help
And each one of us cares."

The nurses turned to smile,
Let me know they were there
Tho they had their own patients,
Providing comfort and care.

They wake each morning
With their lives all their own.
As they enter this building
Their senses they hone.

They tune into the needs
Of those who come for meds
Or are terribly sick,
Whether in chairs or in beds.

Some may work for hours,
Never taking a needed break.
Lunch is non-existent,
A restroom they might make.

For it is their quest
To make us all well,
Knowing what they put in us
Wreaks havoc and hell.

Cancer is relentless
And the patients keep coming.
They make room for more
And keep the place humming.

These dedicated individuals
Who give up their days
Make such a huge impact
In oh so many ways.

Had I not become ill
I never would have met
These wonderful caregivers.
I am forever in their debt.

ABOUT THE AUTHOR

Born and raised in Connecticut, Pam Lacko currently lives in Simsbury with her husband, Jeff; two children, Rebecca and Mathew; and their two golden retrievers. At the age of 47, she was diagnosed with Stage IIB Ovarian Cancer but managed to maintain her daily involvement in all aspects of life. Three years later she continues to run a successful computer-consulting business and donates her spare time to the Simsbury Chamber of Commerce, the Simsbury school system, and cancer-relief efforts in the area. One of the latter is an annual "Women Only, Bad Golfing Encouraged" golf tournament benefiting the American Cancer Society. She was recently given the Simsbury Hometown Hero award.

Soon after her diagnosis, Pam began to write a blog documenting her experiences with surgeries, treatments and emotional reactions. That blog has now become this book, which she hopes will help those experiencing significant medical events such as cancer and encourage them to smile a bit.

This book is set in Garamond Premier Pro, which had its genesis in 1988 when type-designer Robert Slimbach visited the Plantin-Moretus Museum in Antwerp, Belgium, to study its collection of Claude Garamond's metal punches and typefaces. During the mid-fifteen hundreds, Garamond—a Parisian punch-cutter—produced a refined array of book types that combined an unprecedented degree of balance and elegance, for centuries standing as the pinnacle of beauty and practicality in type-founding. Slimbach has created an entirely new interpretation based on Garamond's designs and on comparable italics cut by Robert Granjon, Garamond's contemporary.

To order additional copies of this book
or other Antrim House titles, contact the publisher at

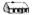

Antrim House
21 Goodrich Rd., Simsbury, CT 06070
860.217.0023, AntrimHouse@comcast.net
or the house website (www.AntrimHouseBooks.com).

•

On the house website
are sample poems, upcoming events,
and a "seminar room" featuring supplemental biography,
notes, images, poems, reviews, and
writing suggestions.